# WELFARE CONDITIONALITY

Welfare conditionality has become an idea of global significance in recent years. A 'hot topic' in North America, Australia, and across Europe, it has been linked to austerity politics and the rise of foodbanks and destitution. In the Global South, where publicly funded welfare protection systems are often absent, conditional approaches have become a key tool employed by organisations pursuing human development goals.

The essence of welfare conditionality lies in requirements for people to behave in prescribed ways in order to access cash benefits or other welfare support. These conditions are typically enforced through benefit 'sanctions' of various kinds, reflecting a new vision of 'welfare', focused more on promoting 'pro-social' behaviour than on protecting people against classic 'social risks' like unemployment.

This new book in Routledge's *Key Ideas* series charts the rise of behavioural conditionality in welfare systems across the globe, its appeal to politicians of Right and Left, and its application to a growing range of social problems. Crucially it explores why, in the context of widespread use of conditional approaches as well as apparently strong public support, both the *efficacy* and the *ethics* of welfare conditionality remain so controversial. As such, *Welfare Conditionality* is essential reading for students, researchers and commentators in social and public policy, as well as those designing and implementing welfare policies.

**Beth Watts** is Senior Research Fellow at the Institute for Social Policy, Housing and Equalities Research (I-SPHERE), Heriot-Watt University. She has a background in political and moral philosophy, and is interested in the application of philosophical tools in social and housing policy analysis. Beth completed her PhD comparing homelessness policy in Scotland and Ireland in 2013 at the University of York, and has previously worked at the Young Foundation, the Joseph Rowntree Foundation, and Shelter.

**Suzanne Fitzpatrick** is Professor of Housing and Social Policy and Director of I-SPHERE, Heriot-Watt University. She completed her PhD on youth homelessness at the University of Glasgow in 1998. Suzanne held various posts in the Department of Urban Studies at the University of Glasgow until 2003, when she was appointed the Joseph Rowntree Professor of Housing Policy and Director of the Centre for Housing Policy at the University of York. Suzanne has a background in law, and specialises in research on homelessness and housing exclusion.

# KEY IDEAS

Series Editor: Peter Hamilton

Designed to compliment the successful *Key Sociologists*, this series covers the main concepts, issues, debates, and controversies in sociology and the social sciences. The series aims to provide authoritative essays on central topics of social science, such as community, power, work, sexuality, inequality, benefits and ideology, class, and family. Books adopt a strong 'individual' line, as critical essays rather than literature surveys, offering lively and original treatments of their subject matter. The books will be useful to students and teachers of sociology, political science, economics, psychology, philosophy, and geography.

www.routledge.com/Key-Ideas/book-series/SE0058

**Knowledge – second edition**
**Is Knowledge Power?**
*Marian Adolf and Nico Stehr*

**Sexuality – fourth edition**
*Jeffrey Weeks*

**Social Capital – third edition**
*John Field*

**Patriarchy**
*Pavla Miller*

**Populism: An Introduction**
*Manuel Anselmi*

**Community – third edition**
*Gerard Delanty*

**Welfare Conditionality**
*Beth Watts and Suzanne Fitzpatrick*

# WELFARE CONDITIONALITY

*Beth Watts and Suzanne Fitzpatrick*

Routledge
Taylor & Francis Group
LONDON AND NEW YORK

First published 2018
by Routledge
2 Park Square, Milton Park, Abingdon, Oxon OX14 4RN

and by Routledge
711 Third Avenue, New York, NY 10017

*Routledge is an imprint of the Taylor & Francis Group, an informa business*



*British Library Cataloguing-in-Publication Data*
A catalogue record for this book is available from the British Library

*Library of Congress Cataloging-in-Publication Data*
Names: Watts, Beth, author. | Fitzpatrick, Suzanne, 1969- author.
Title: Welfare conditionality / Beth Watts and Suzanne Fitzpatrick.
Description: 1st Edition. | New York : Routledge, 2018. | Series: Key ideas | Includes bibliographical references and index.
Identifiers: LCCN 2017059143| ISBN 9781138119901 (hardback) | ISBN 9781138119918 (pbk.) | ISBN 9781315652047 (ebook)
Subjects: LCSH: Public welfare. | Social policy.
Classification: LCC HV31 .W38 2018 | DDC 361.6/1–dc23
LC record available at https://lccn.loc.gov/2017059143

ISBN: 978-1-138-11990-1 (hbk)
ISBN: 978-1-138-11991-8 (pbk)
ISBN: 978-1-315-65204-7 (ebk)

Typeset in Bembo
by Swales & Willis Ltd, Exeter, Devon, UK

# CONTENTS

# ACKNOWLEDGEMENTS

We are very grateful for Professor Mark Stephens' and Professor Sarah Johnsen's detailed and thoughtful comments on draft chapters. We would like to record our particular thanks to our dear friend and inspiring colleague, Professor Glen Bramley. His supportive reflections and sharp insights on the full draft manuscript provided the challenge and reassurance we needed to get 'over the line'.

Our thanks are also owed to Professor Volker Busch-Geertsema, Ruth Owen, Maria Jose Aldanas and Sarah Coupechoux for their help in resolving a tricky query. We would further like to record our gratitude to Professor Ruth Grant and Dr Stuart White for their helpful correspondence during our time working on the book, which we drew upon in developing our ideas.

The support of the Economic and Social Research Council (ESRC) under grant number ES/K002163/2 is gratefully acknowledged, with thanks also to all of our colleagues on the Welfare Conditionality project led by Professor Peter Dwyer at the University of York. Any errors and all opinions remain ours alone.

# 1

# INTRODUCTION

The use of increasingly conditional forms of welfare is widely understood to be a relatively recent and radical shift in the nature of social policy across advanced economies. Usually dated from the 1990s, 'welfare conditionality' has been described as reflecting a 'new vision of the welfare state' (Watson, 2015, p.646), focused less on protecting individuals from the risks associated with market forces or smoothing income over the life course (Hill, 2014) and instead 'intent on converting the welfare benefits system into a lever for changing behaviour' (Rodger, 2008, p.87). The intensification of conditionality in Western welfare systems, and in particular in the UK, is the main focus of this book. But an adequate account of these developments requires framing within the much-longer-term history of welfare provision being deployed as a mechanism of 'social control' to shape the behaviour of those who avail themselves of state-funded support. It must also make connection with the rolling out of conditional forms of welfare in the very different social, economic and policy contexts of the Global South.

The starting point for our analysis is that access to welfare provision is necessarily structured by legally or administratively defined boundaries, requirements and rules – in other words, 'conditions'. Typically, claimants must share relevant information with 'street-level bureaucrats' (Lipsky, 1980), attend interviews and respond to letters (Griggs and Evans, 2010). Whether cooperation with these processes will afford claimants access to the welfare benefit or good sought will further depend on their meeting some combination of conditions concerning their *status* (are they eligible based on criteria such as citizenship, local residency and age bracket?), *need* (do they require assistance because they are sick, disabled, homeless, unemployed or on a low income?), and *conduct* (have they behaved in the ways required to access the benefit or good in question?). The requirement for claimants to meet at least some minimum relevant criteria is thus inescapable, even in the case of so-called 'universal' benefits (Spicker, 2005; Clasen and Clegg, 2007; Dwyer, 2010).

These conditions need not, of course, include conduct elements, and can instead be limited to the domains of status and need just noted. However, it has long been recognised that welfare provision, whether or not it includes explicit behavioural conditions, will have *behavioural effects*. The unintended 'perverse' incentives or 'moral hazard' associated with welfare systems is held responsible in some quarters for creating a dependent 'underclass' unwilling and/or unable to work (Mead, 1986, 1997; Murray, 1984, 1990, 1994; Dunn, 2014; Perkins, 2016), with concerns about such an underclass not limited to the political Right (Field, 1989; Wilson, 1997). Writing from a very different perspective, and reflecting a well-established tradition of applying Foucauldian insights to social policy concerns, Hartley Dean (1991) argues that the very act of claiming social security benefits 'brings into play an intricate set of rules of entitlement which announce the duties of the claimant as a citizen and which, by tests and obstacles so imposed upon the claimant, bear upon him/her with "normalising" effect' (pp.42–43). Welfare policies are, from this perspective, intrinsically *socially controlling* (Chriss, 2007), in that provision of goods and services by the state or other welfare providers inevitably creates an 'incentive architecture' (Grant, 2006) that shapes, moulds and constrains the choices people make.

That welfare policy *explicitly* and *intentionally* influences behaviour through conduct-related conditions is also not a new phenomenon. The historical antecedents of such behavioural conditionality in the UK are usually traced back to the emergence of and subsequent reforms to the Poor Laws (both the 'old' Elizabeth Poor Law, and in particular the 1834 'new' Poor Law), which sought in their different ways to both relieve poverty and to deter reliance on that relief. The new Poor Laws marked a key attempt to encourage self-reliance through the principle of 'less eligibility', which prescribed that conditions in workhouses had to be worse than conditions available outside to deter the claiming of poor relief (Mitchell Dean, 1991). John Stuart Mill described the problem facing social reformers in the mid nineteenth century as 'how to give the greatest amount of needful help with the smallest encouragement to undue reliance on it' (Mill, 1848, cited in Goodin, 1985, p.28). Hartley Dean (1991) traces the origins of behavioural conditionality back even further, pointing to Edward III's attempts in the mid fourteenth century to ensure that 'valiant beggars . . . may be compelled to labour for their necessary living' and commenting that since that time 'the state has continued by various means of repression to attempt to compel those who are capable of productive work to "labour for their necessary living"' (p.43).

Bringing us back to the modern era, numerous commentators have emphasised that the foundations of the post-war UK welfare state were not laid on the promise of *universal* and *unconditional* social rights. On the contrary, the principle of work-related conditionality was integral to the thinking of its architects – Beveridge, Temple and Tawney (Deacon, 1994; Freud, 2007; Daguerre and Etherington, 2014). Certainly, the formative Beveridge (1942) report made clear that after a certain period, cash benefits should be conditional on attendance at a work or a training centre. Scholars differ, however, in the extent to which they see the current system of welfare conditionality and benefit sanctions in the UK as in the spirit of the post-welfare settlement (Freud, 2007), as a gross exaggeration of it (Dwyer, 2010) or as a manifestation of its intrinsic flaws and contradictions present from the very beginning (Philips, 2000).

Likewise, there has been much attention paid to the 'activation turn' across Continental Europe since the 1990s (Eichorst and Konle-Seidl, 2008; Keune and Serrano, 2013), intrinsic to which was an increased emphasis on conditional forms of welfare (Clasen and Clegg, 2006). However, this movement has longer-term roots going back at least as far as mid twentieth century Sweden, where successive administrations sought to balance social democratic ideals of equality, solidarity and social protection with the desire to maintain full employment and the need to ensure economic competitiveness and growth (Bonoli, 2010). Denmark's 'flexicurity state' is now seen to represent the apotheosis of this active labour market approach (Brodkin and Larsen, 2013), with its emphasis on enabling citizens to adjust to changing labour market trends, while maintaining their security and wellbeing, through retraining and human capital development programmes. German reforms to unemployment benefits in the mid 2000s (the 'Hartz reforms') drew on developments in Denmark, the Netherlands and the UK (Bonoli, 2010), the latter of which had taken lessons from the US's 'work first' approach, with its much stronger ideological commitment to work as a moral duty and conception of welfare dependency as a personal failing (Murray, 1994; Mead, 1997).

Placed in such historical context, it is clear that the recent intensification of behavioural conditionality through the 'tools' of welfare provision in the UK and elsewhere must be seen as the latest chapter in the ebb and flow of more and less 'activating', 'responsibilising' and 'disciplinary' manifestations of welfare states (Brodkin and Larsen, 2013). Nonetheless, while perhaps not quite the fundamental departure that some of its critics appear to suggest, this 'conditional turn' in welfare systems has elicited great interest and significant controversy with good reason, given the sharp expansion in both its reach and impact.

## The broadening and deepening of welfare conditionality

The controversy surrounding recent intensification of behavioural conditionality in Western democracies relates in part to the *increased severity* of the sanctions applied to those whose conduct fails to conform to requirements. In the UK, there is now provision for full removal of benefits for up to three years from unemployed people who fail to meet work-related activity requirements (Watts et al., 2014), while in the US immediate full-family sanctions operate in a variety of states (Casey, 2010; Mead, 2011). The stringency of conditions and severity of sanctions has also increased in Canada and New Zealand in recent years, and in many developed welfare states claimants are required to accept job offers at much lower rates of pay and in different occupations than their previous employment, as well as at considerable distances and travel times from their home (Langenbucher, 2015). While sanctions tend to be less severe in north-western European countries, there has nonetheless been a tendency for these to be strengthened in recent years (Langenbucher, 2015). For example, in Germany the 2003–05 'Hartz' reforms introduced significantly more onerous obligations on unemployed people than had previously been the case, backed by stronger sanctioning mechanisms involving benefit reductions and suspensions of up to 12 weeks (Jacobi and Kluve, 2007; Langenbucher, 2015; Bothfeld and Rosenthal, 2017). In the UK at least, evidence is accumulating that the intensification of benefit sanctions is associated, for example, with the recent sharp escalation in the use of foodbanks (Sosenko et al., 2013; Lambie-Mumford, 2014), as well as with heightened risks of absolute destitution (Fitzpatrick et al., 2016) and homelessness (Batty et al., 2015).

Moreover, extensive evidence from the UK, US and elsewhere has indicated the *disproportionate effect* of work-related welfare sanctions on particular sections of the population including young people (Pavetti et al., 2003; Peters and Joyce, 2006; Watts et al., 2014; de Vries et al., 2017), homeless people (Oakley, 2014; Reeve, 2017), and ethnic minority communities (Peters and Joyce, 2006; Dwyer, 2009; Schram et al., 2009; de Vries et al., 2017), as well as a variety of other groups such as those with mental health problems or low levels of qualifications, work experience, literacy or numeracy (Bonjour et al., 2001; Pavetti et al., 2003; Peters and Joyce, 2006; Fording et al., 2013; Church Poverty Action Group et al., 2015). This has served to heighten disquiet about both the fairness and the impacts of such sanctions (Griggs and Evans, 2010; Watts et al., 2014; Reeve and Loopstra, 2017).

There has also been an expansion in the *range of welfare claimants* affected by behavioural conditionality. Benefits for sick and disabled people now embrace substantial elements of conditionality in a wide range of developed economies, spanning the UK and Australia, as well as Scandinavian and Northern European countries, albeit that the emphasis on accompanying supports tends to be stronger in Continental Europe, with a willingness to employ sanctions stronger in the

Anglosphere countries (Geiger, 2017). Lone parents, too, have been brought within the ambit of conditionality, with almost all Organisation for Economic Co-operation and Development (OECD) countries applying a 'work test' to this group when the parent's youngest child reaches a certain age (under one in some US and Canadian states, though usually higher in Europe and Australasia) (Finn and Gloster, 2010). The UK was relatively late in applying work-related conditionality to this group, but since 2008 incremental reforms have brought increasingly higher numbers of lone parents, with ever-younger children, inside the conditionality regime (Whitworth and Griggs, 2013; Johnsen, 2016). In the US, lone parents have long since been key targets of conditionality, particularly since the introduction of 'Temporary Assistance for Needy Families' in the mid-1990s, which explicitly aimed to end the dependence of recipient households (largely Hispanic or African American single mothers) on such benefits via work-tests and time limits on assistance (Falk, 2016). A further frontier is now being crossed, in the UK at least, with the extension of welfare conditionality beyond those who are unemployed to those in low-paid or part-time work. The phasing in of the 'Universal Credit' regime, which combines a range of previously separate working-age benefits, means that those whose weekly gross earnings fall short of a 'conditionality threshold' will be expected to meet the threshold by working more hours and/or increasing their pay rate to avoid sanctions on their in-work benefits (Dwyer and Wright, 2014).

There is also a broadening in the *range of welfare spheres* within which conditional approaches have been introduced (Watts et al., 2014). This includes the housing realm, with social tenants in England and parts of Australia, for example, who previously could have expected open-ended lifetime tenancies, now offered more conditional fixed-term contracts, with renewal procedures potentially taking into account income, employment status and various aspects of behaviour (Fitzpatrick and Pawson, 2014; Fitzpatrick and Watts, 2017). In the related field of homelessness, too, there has been a (highly controversial) trend across the Global North towards increasingly conditional offers of support alongside enforcement and other 'interventionist' policies which seek to alter the behaviour and lifestyle of rough sleepers (Mitchell, 1997; Amster, 2003; DeVerteuil, May and von Mahs, 2009;

Johnsen and Fitzpatrick, 2010; Whiteford, 2010; Parsell, 2011; Bowpitt et al., 2014; Watts et al., 2017). Relevant examples are to be found too in the health, education and child protection spheres, especially in the Global South, where 'conditional cash transfers' often seek to incentivise parents to enrol their children in school and have them immunised (Bastagli, 2009; Barrientos, 2011; Pellerano and Barca, 2014). Australia has pioneered a range of child welfare-focused conditionality measures, including highly controversial 'compulsory income management' policies which disproportionately impact on Indigenous claimants (Taylor et al., 2016). Proposals to reform social security benefits as a lever to force people to address drug or alcohol addictions (e.g. through drug testing), and other health and 'lifestyle' issues like obesity, have also emerged across the Global North in recent years, including in the US, Canada, the UK and Australia, though in many cases they have not yet progressed into law given their highly controversial reception and concerns about their likely efficacy (Wincup, 2014; Black, 2016; Pérez-Muñoz, 2017).

## Conditionality, austerity and public opinion

A key reason why the current 'conditionality turn' in welfare might be viewed as particularly controversial is its association with post-Global Financial Crisis (GFC) 'austerity politics'. Theories of policy change generally emphasise the importance of path dependence and incremental change, with 'destabilising large exogenous shocks' such as the financial crisis understood to create potential windows of opportunity for more radical change (Hudson and Lowe, 2009; Farnsworth and Irving, 2011; Vis et al., 2011). It has been hypothesised, on the one hand, that the GFC would lead to a renewal of support for and appreciation of the value of social spending as reliance on the labour market to provide security and welfare became less tenable, and on the other, that it would lead to a greater emphasis on active labour market policies (including behavioural conditionality) and efforts to reduce public spending in response to the fiscal crisis (Vis et al., 2011; Marchal et al., 2014; see also Farnsworth and Irving, 2011). In reality, the response to the GFC seems, at least initially, to have been surprisingly similar across a range of European countries and the US, with initial support to banks followed by macro-economic policies which 'upheld and expanded rather than retrenched welfare programmes' (Vis et al., 2011, p.339). An austerity-driven retrenchment phase then ensued in most instances, albeit that the nature and extent of these governmental bids to significantly reduce public expenditure varied, with hostile public opinion offering resistance in a number of countries (Kersbergen et al., 2014; Vis et al., 2011).

The connection to be made between austerity politics and behavioural conditionality may seem self-evident, with intensified conditionality offering policy makers a win/win tool: either claimants comply with behavioural requirements and (assuming at least some degree of effectiveness of these kinds of approaches for the time being) make less use of welfare benefits and services, thus reducing public expenditure, or they do not, in which case sanctions and exclusions from these services nevertheless accrue savings (Adler and Terum, 2017). The US experience, and some recent work in the UK, certainly demonstrates the significance of these measures in diverting substantial numbers of claimants away from welfare programmes via the 'hassle factor' associated with making and maintaining a claim, regardless of whether those affected subsequently find paid employment (Finn and Goodship, 2014; Mead, 2014; Loopstra et al., 2015a).

However, austerity and conditionality are perhaps less closely aligned than might initially be assumed (Adler and Terum, 2017). For a start, substantial pushes towards behavioural forms of conditionality occurred in the UK and Germany, and certainly in the US and Sweden, well before the GFC. Moreover, a core contribution of comparative research in this field has been to demonstrate the distinct varieties of active labour market policies pursued in different countries, some of which combine stringent conditionality with heavy investment in employment support and other 'enabling' elements, such as childcare provision, as well as high 'replacement rates' (i.e. the extent to which out-of-work benefits replace the level of income received when employed) (Eichhorst and Konle-Seidl, 2008). Denmark is archetypical of this model, while the US and UK, in stark contrast, combine strict conditionality with much lower replacement ratios and weaker human capital investment (Eichhorst and Konle-Seidl, 2008; Langenbucher, 2015).

It is also worth noting that, in cases where decision-makers and political elites *are* intent on welfare retrenchment and reducing social spending as their overriding aims, increased behavioural conditionality is unlikely to represent the most straightforward means to these ends. Indeed, armed with the necessary political will, alongside the required public appetite or indifference, it is much easier and cheaper to simply remove or severely restrict the welfare entitlements of entire sections of the population and/or to impose cuts on other kinds of social spending (for example, grants to local government or the third sector). There is certainly plenty of evidence of these types of policies post the GFC. From 2009, cuts in benefit levels were pursued aggressively in Ireland, one of the countries first and worst hit by the GFC, with single unemployed people – especially young people – and one-parent families particularly badly hit (Keane et al., 2014). Cuts to unemployment benefit levels and/or the duration of entitlements have also been pursued in Germany, the Netherlands and Denmark since the financial crisis (Kersbergen et al., 2014).

In the UK, too, the period post 2010 has seen very substantial cuts in the coverage and generosity of working-age benefits, with younger people, larger families and various migrant groups worst affected (Hills, 2014; Fitzpatrick et al., 2017). All of those entitled to working-age benefits will also see their entitlements progressively whittled down over the coming years as payment rates are 'frozen' in cash terms rather than rising with inflation (Beatty and Fothergill, 2016b). This ongoing benefits freeze is associated with far larger savings to the public purse (an estimated £3.5 billion in 2019/20 alone and £10 billion over five years) than any direct reductions in welfare expenditure attributable to the ramping up of the sanction regime (an estimated £135 million in 2015) (Department for Work and Pensions, 2015; National Audit Office, 2016). Indeed, the UK's National Audit Office has warned that the cost of administering benefit conditionality and the knock-on impact on other public services may well mean that the sanctions regime *costs* money, rather than saving it (NAO, 2016). All of these benefit cuts have gone alongside swingeing cuts to local authority funding (Hastings et al., 2015).

Perhaps the most significant factor casting doubt on any *necessary* association between welfare conditionality and austerity agendas is the use of behavioural conditionality (in the form of 'conditional cash transfers') in less economically developed countries to promote engagement with health services and education. In these contexts, such policy developments appear to be part of an attempt to *establish* social protection systems, rather than *retrench* them (Bastagli, 2009; Fiszbein et al., 2009).

Nonetheless, though 'gentler breeds' of conditionality are documented in the literature, it is clear that a consensus in favour of behavioural conditionality *has* combined in many developed economies with declining levels of welfare generosity and coverage, together amounting to a highly significant shift in the character of welfare systems. Certainly, Right-wing critics of Western post-war welfare states often view the intensification of conditionality, alongside cuts in the level and scope of entitlements, as a necessary corrective to what they see as the past profligacy of over-generous benefits which damaged work incentives and created a dependent 'underclass' with 'employment resistant personalities' (Mead, 1997; Philips, 2000; Dunn, 2014; Perkins, 2016).

It has also been argued, especially in the UK and US, that there is public support for benefit conditionality, aligned to a more general hardening of attitudes towards unemployed people (Dwyer, 2000; Taylor Gooby, 2005; Bastagli, 2009; Sage, 2012), allowing proponents of these approaches to claim a democratic mandate. Public attitudes are, however, often complex and ambivalent on such matters, with evidence from the UK and elsewhere also pointing to enduring popular support for the welfare state (Vis et al., 2011; Hudson et al., 2016). That said, there is a plausible case to be made that public support for behavioural conditionality may be increasing in countries that have pursued this trajectory of reform precisely because such conditional and targeted approaches undermine support for 'collective notions of fairness [and] social cohesion' (Sage, 2012; see also Larsen, 2006). Indeed, conditionality has been argued to be one manifestation of a divisive politics of resentment that (mis)uses the concept of fairness to fuel reactionary populism and 'anti-welfare' discourses (Hoggett et al., 2013).

This is linked to more fundamental political economy critiques that accuse those promoting conditional forms of welfare as misrepresenting 'structural' problems of economic and industrial decline as instead attributable to 'psychological deficits' amongst the people directly affected (Friedli and Stearn, 2015), and then adding insult to injury by impoverishing the very same people via benefit cuts (Watson, 2015). In the UK, this case has been particularly powerfully argued in recent years by Christina Beatty and Steve Fothergill (2013, 2016a, 2016b), who in a broad-ranging overview contended that:

> The [UK] Treasury has misdiagnosed high welfare spending as the result of inadequate work incentives and has too often blamed individuals for their own predicament, whereas in fact a large part of the bill is rooted in job destruction extending back decades ... The welfare reforms implemented since 2010, and strengthened since the 2015 general election, hit the poorest places hardest. In effect, communities in older industrial Britain are being meted out punishment in the form of welfare cuts for the destruction wrought to their industrial base.
>
> *(Beatty and Fothergill, 2016a, p.2)*

## Conditionality and social control

At its heart, behavioural conditionality is a form of social control – an exercise of power (Bachrach and Baratz, 1963; Lukes, 2005) – targeting claimants and recipients of publicly-funded welfare programmes. More specifically, it is a form of *coercive* power (Lukes, 2005), which uses the threat of deprivation (of welfare goods) to achieve behavioural change on the part of those in need of them (Watts et al., 2017; Johnsen et al., forthcoming). Attitudes to the ethical dilemmas and practical questions that this raises are likely to be rooted in the underlying values (Haidt and Graham, 2007) and view of society (Chriss, 2007) to which one subscribes, and in particular whether an essentially 'consensus' or 'conflict' model is seen to be most persuasive.

According to *consensus* theories, society can be thought of as an organic system held together by functional elements, including shared norms and values that maintain order and stability (Chriss, 2007). These norms emerge because they serve some useful purpose and are then passed on through tradition, imitation and authority. On this view, mechanisms of social control help secure the 'public good' of social solidarity and social order – necessary conditions for people to achieve their goals (Durkheim, 1893/1984; Tonnies, 1955). It has been argued that a perceived crisis in traditional community- and family-based forms of social control, and failure of the 'organic' modes of control to emerge in their place (Chriss, 2007), has led to greater reliance on the 'specialised application of rules and sanctions by designated agents of the state' (Horwitz, 1990, p.2). On this view, the disciplinary/controlling nature of welfare provision is a necessary response to the crises of socialisation and community, resonating with 'new communitarian' thinking (e.g. Etzioni, 1994, 1997; Selbourne, 1994; Dwyer, 2000) and concerns about 'dependency culture' cited above, likely to particularly appeal to those placing high value on norms of authority and ingroup loyalty (Haidt and Graham, 2007).

In sharp contrast, *conflict* theories of society interpret social order as maintained by advantaged groups in pursuit of their own interests, rather than in service of general societal benefit (Chriss, 2007). Norms, laws, policies and the whole gamut of social control mechanisms are thus viewed as positioning the non-privileged as deviant, criminal, insane, indolent or simply undeserving. Fed by 'a growing disillusionment with the achievements of state welfare' in improving the conditions of disadvantaged groups (Higgins, 1980, p.3), this kind of perspective has challenged the status of the welfare state as a 'purely humanitarian enterprise' (p.21), casting doubt on claims that 'the social assistance programmes of the welfare state are best seen as devices to protect the vulnerable and dependent beneficiaries' (Goodin, p.145). Rather, the welfare state is viewed as a monolithic and oppressive set of institutions; a 'means by which the ruling class could avoid the revolutionary dangers inherent in increasing alienation and provide a disciplined, effective and healthy workforce' (Corrigan and Leonard, cited in Higgins, 1980, p.13).

While the consensus model has increasingly been seen as simplistic and naive, conflict models of society have also been criticised as crude, and discredited due to their association with Marxism (Higgins, 1980). Post-structuralist perspectives, for example, highlight the potential for resistance on the part of both welfare 'agents' and welfare 'users' (Barnes and Prior, 2009). Higgins (1980) contends that understandings of social policy based on conflict models tend to homogenize and oversimplify the functions of social policies and the welfare state, and read the *intent* of policy makers by looking only at the *effects* of policies, rather than exploring the actual motivations and interests of specific actors – the controlling effects of certain policies may or may not have been the conscious intention of the policy makers who designed them, or the administrators who implement them.

This sort of perspective complements the more recent contribution to welfare state theory offered by Clarke (2004), who argues that 'welfare states' are not 'coherent single entities' but 'compound institutional formations' subject to 'divergent pressures' (p.19). As such, welfare states may be 'internally contradictory' (p.19) or 'more than one thing at once' (p.2). Other scholars have similarly posited that welfare states and social policies – and those administering them – are likely to pursue a plurality of (sometimes contradictory) objectives. Writing from a political philosophy perspective, a range of authors contend that values themselves are plural (e.g. need and desert, equality and liberty) and potentially in conflict (Berlin, 1969; Miller, 1999; Ignatieff, 2000). Moral psychologists have empirically mapped this value pluralism, identifying five 'moral foundations' (Harm/Care, Fairness/Reciprocity, Ingroup/Loyalty, Authority/Respect, and Purity/Sanctity) reflected in public attitudes globally, with variation in the level of commitment to these different values not just in different world regions, but also *within* Western democracies (Graham et al., 2011). Hoggett (2006), focusing on public bureaucracies and policy implementation, argues that these institutions 'contain' anxieties, contradictions and unresolved issues passed on to them by higher tiers of government.

If these latter analyses are accepted, neither the consensus or conflict models of society appear adequate: instead society might be seen as open and pluralistic (Jones et al., 1978), characterised by multiple ongoing conflicts between different groups, with varying levels of power, and distinctive value bases. Welfare and social policies may be understood as both a 'humanitarian enterprise' *and* 'mechanisms of social control', with the precise balance between these characterisations shifting back and forth over time, and varying between different welfare spheres and systems.

This standpoint is consistent with an emergent literature within applied areas of social policy that demonstrates potentially complex and contradictory motivations for, and outcomes of, policy and practice. Pheonix (2008), for instance, talks of 'coercive welfare' in the context of state responses to prostitution, and Johnsen and Fitzpatrick (2010) of 'coercive care' in the context of responses to rough sleepers and those engaged in street activities (see also Flint, 2009a). This indicates that dichotomous, all-encompassing characterisations of welfare policies as either punitive or caring, empowering or disempowering, disciplinary or ameliorative, are unlikely to be helpful, with attention needing to be paid to the specifics of both policy mechanisms and contexts, and their empirical outcomes, to make fair and well-grounded normative assessments.

## This book

The debates on welfare conditionality reviewed above pose a series of theoretical, empirical and normative questions. How might we best conceptualise welfare conditionality, and appropriately contextualise it in relation to other policy tools and interventions that seek to change the behaviour of welfare claimants? How convincing are the assumptions regarding behavioural responses implied by these conditional policies? What values underpin the pursuit or rejection of behavioural conditionality as a legitimate welfare policy tool? Are these values and ethical positions defensible and coherent? Are the aims, motivations and ethical positions of policy makers and service providers employing conduct conditionality consistent across countries, areas of welfare and distinct intervention models? What do we know about the practical outcomes and impacts of these conditional forms of welfare?

This book aims to address these questions by mapping out the key theories and empirical evidence relevant to understanding and evaluating conditional welfare policies. The origins of the book lie in a major international evidence, policy and normative review undertaken as part of a five-year research programme, *Welfare conditionality: sanctions support and behaviour change* (see www.welfareconditionality.ac.uk), funded by the UK's Economic and Social Research Council (ESRC). As such, the starting point of our analysis is the specific evolution and impact of welfare conditionality in the UK case, but we place this national 'story' in the context of parallel developments in other developed-economy welfare systems, and also make relevant links with the extension of conditional forms of welfare across many parts of the Global South. Like the project itself, the book focuses on those aspects of welfare systems and conditionality which are most likely to affect economically and socially disadvantaged sections of the population. This includes, in particular, means-tested cash transfer programmes of various kinds, especially for working-age populations, but also conditionality in the realm of housing, homelessness and anti-social behaviour programmes. As we will see over the course of the book, these are also the domains within which welfare conditionality is most likely to take a 'harder' sanction-based form. We do, however, consider some especially relevant examples of conditionality in, for example, the health and educational spheres, particularly where these measures are related to cash-based sanctions and incentives.

Chapter 2 of the book sets the *context for conditionality* by considering other key parameters on which welfare systems vary, such as the generosity of benefit levels and the legal basis on which they are distributed. Chapter 3 then reviews in detail the *techniques of conditionality*, including the substantive behavioural requirements, monitoring and surveillance processes, and sanctions and incentives applied. Chapter 4 focuses on the *subjects of conditionality*, and explores why and how conditional approaches have been targeted at particular groups of welfare recipients, focusing on unemployed people, young people, sick and disabled people, families with children, social tenants and those experiencing homelessness. Chapter 5 examines the *impacts of conditionality*, setting the evidence on the outcomes, effectiveness and costs of conditional welfare techniques, and any unintended consequences, in the context of the behavioural assumptions that appear to underpin the 'theory of change' implicit in these models. It also highlights alternative methods for achieving desired forms of behavioural change. Chapter 6 explores the *ethics of conditionality*, interrogating how this stance may be supported and contested from a range of normative perspectives, including that of 'human rights', 'citizenship', 'utilitarianism', 'contractualism', 'communitarianism', 'paternalism' and 'social justice'. Chapter 7 concludes the book by offering readers a framework within which to *assess the efficacy and ethical legitimacy* of conditional approaches to welfare provision and practice.

# 2

# THE CONTEXT FOR CONDITIONALITY

This chapter places welfare conditionality in its broader policy context by considering other dimensions on which welfare provision may vary. Specifically, it locates behavioural conditionality as one among several potential forms of welfare *targeting*, and differentiates targeting from two other conceptually distinct aspects of welfare provision – its *generosity* and whether it is provided on the basis of *entitlement* or discretion.

The key point is that *who* gets access to welfare (targeting) is a conceptually separate question from *how much* of that welfare they get (generosity), which in turn is a quite distinct matter from the *legal basis of their claim* to that welfare (entitlement or discretion) (see also Clasen and Clegg, 2007; Dean, 2002). Understanding these distinctions and their interrelationship is fundamental to appreciating the aims, significance and impact of specific conditional welfare techniques, to which we turn our attention in Chapter 3.

## Targeting

A broad contrast is often drawn between 'universal' and 'selective' forms of welfare provision (for example, Dean, 2002; Gugushvili and Hirsch,

2014). In Esping-Andersen's (1990) classic 'welfare regime' typology, 'social democratic' systems (such as in Sweden) are said to give rise to low levels of poverty and inequality in part because they offer more universalistic and generous benefits, in contrast to the targeted, means-tested allowances characteristic of 'liberal' regimes of English speaking countries. The distribution of particular welfare goods – cash benefits, housing, education, health – can also be more or less universalistic or selective. Comparative housing studies, for instance, has contrasted the 'universalistic' housing policies, epitomised by Sweden's 'unitary' rental housing market, with the more 'selective' social housing regime found in Anglosphere countries including the UK, but more especially Australia, the US and Canada, wherein much stricter needs and/or means testing is applied in social housing allocation (Bengtsson, 2001). This selectivity or universality in the housing sphere may go with the grain of the broader welfare regime, or cut against it (Stephens and Fitzpatrick, 2007).

It has been argued that universal welfare interventions are more likely than selective ones to attract durable public support and promote social integration, as a less clear dividing line is drawn between 'us' (contributors) and 'them' (recipients) (Korpi and Palme, 1998; Larsen, 2006; Bastagli, 2009, Standing, 2011; Hoggett et al., 2013). Others have disputed the empirical basis of this claimed association between universal benefits and resilience to cutbacks (Kenworthy, 2011), and have also highlighted the potentially regressive distributive effects of 'universal' provision that 'by definition allocate more to the non-poor majority than the poor minority' (Gugushvili and Hirsch, 2014, p.6). It is also worth pointing out that some allegedly 'universal' European welfare systems in fact offered very limited protection for those who did not qualify for contribution-based 'social insurance' benefits, with France, for example, only introducing a 'social assistance' safety net in the 1980s (Clasen and Clegg, 2006).

Nonetheless, the shift to more intensively selective approaches (e.g. from contributory to predominantly means-tested benefits) in the UK and most other European countries in the post-war period has been lamented by many, in large part because of concerns about stigma, low take-up and high administrative costs, as well as potential work disincentives (Gugushvili and Hirsch, 2014). With the exception of housing (often described as the 'wobbly pillar under the welfare state' because provision tends to be dominated by the market; see Torgersen, 1987), there appears to often be stronger public support for universal provision of *in-kind* services, such as health care and education, than for cash transfers (Gugushvili and Hirsch, 2014). The idea of a 'universal basic *income*' has, however, gained support from a range of very different perspectives in recent years, though its application in practice remains rare and small scale (Standing, 2017; Painter and Thoung, 2015).

As noted in the first chapter, however, it is almost inconceivable that any form of welfare entitlement could be truly universal (Dean, 2002). Even the very broadest conceptualisation of 'social citizenship rights' (Dwyer, 2010) or the idea of a 'universal basic income' (Standing, 2017) implies criteria regarding who is recognised as a member of the relevant 'political community' against whom such rights can be claimed (see Miller, 1999). It is therefore most relevant to focus on the nature and breadth of the criteria that delineate access to different forms of welfare provision. It is helpful to distinguish between three types of conditions which can be used to target welfare goods and services (see also Clasen and Clegg, 2007 for a slightly different formulation):

1. Conditions of **status**, i.e. being in the right 'community' or 'universe' to be potentially eligible for receipt of the good/service in question. Frequently-used markers of status in welfare provision include: *citizenship* (with migrant groups often excluded from full and sometimes any access to welfare support); *residency* (living in or having connections to the local or national jurisdiction providing the welfare); *demographic characteristics* (such as being the relevant age, e.g. for pension provision).
2. Conditions of **need**, relating to the specific reason for the claimant's requirement for assistance, e.g. being sick, unemployed, disabled, homeless, having caring responsibilities or having a low income. Such assessments of need can be *categorical* (do they have the relevant need in question, or not), or based on a *threshold* (are they sufficiently 'in need' to access support).
3. Conditions of **conduct**, which specify behavioural conditions that determine either initial access (important examples of such *retrospective conditionality* include the contributions requirements for

social insurance benefits, and the widespread restriction in access to unemployment benefits for those who are deemed to have 'voluntarily' given up work) or continued access (the archetypal example of such *ongoing conditionality* being that recipients of out-of-work benefits must actively seek work throughout their claim).

Conditions of conduct are thus only one criterion used to broker access to welfare provision and, as argued by Adler and Terum (2017), the extent and nature of targeting, including with regard to behavioural conditionality, is not necessarily related to welfare regime type. Policy makers across regime types may trade different forms of targeting off against each other, in the context of heavily constrained public budgets. For example, they may elect to expand the 'universe' of people potentially eligible for a benefit while simultaneously making actual access to this support dependent on higher levels of need or introducing stricter forms of behavioural conditionality. One good example of this is offered by the German 'Hartz' reforms, which simultaneously brought a much wider section of the population within the remit of unemployment benefits (by merging unemployment assistance and social assistance), strengthened the means test specifying access to assistance for this group and introduced stricter conduct conditionality, particularly for young people (Clasen and Clegg, 2007). Another example concerns the shift towards 'free' personal care for older people in Scotland, which expanded the scope of potential eligibility to all those above a certain age, while at the same time significantly increasing the need threshold for access. As Gugushvili and Hirsch (2014) comment, this experience shows that:

> the biggest risk in moving towards universalism [is] a tightening of entitlements that could make poorer people worse off, because they [are] left to fend for themselves until their condition [becomes] very serious.
>
> *(p.51)*

Equally, restrictions in targeting may be pursued across the piece. In the UK, for instance, austerity-driven welfare reforms undertaken by the post 2010 Westminster governments have involved the dramatic ramping up of behavioural conditionality in out-of-work benefits, while at the same time relevant need thresholds have been raised (for example, on disability and sickness benefits), and some groups (defined by migration status or age) have found their eligibility status for particular benefits removed altogether (Barr et al., 2016; Beatty and Fothergill, 2016b; Lupton et al., 2015; Fitzpatrick et al., 2017). Just as important as these structural changes in the targeting of UK benefits, however, has been their declining generosity, the topic to which we now turn.

## Generosity

Welfare provision of all kinds varies in terms of what might be described as 'generosity'. Depending on the nature of the specific welfare good or service in question, issues of generosity may pertain to the *quantity* of cash, goods or services offered; the *duration* for which the relevant benefit, goods or services can be received; and/or their *quality*.

In Esping-Andersen's (1990) terms, welfare benefits may achieve higher or lower levels of 'decommodification' (the degree to which recipients can maintain an acceptable standard of living independently from the labour market), and support greater or lesser degrees of 'stratification' (the extent to which the welfare system sustains work-related status), depending on the level at which they are set. More generous out-of-work benefits will demonstrate a higher replacement rate (the proportion of income in work that is maintained after job loss via the social security system) and/or enable recipients to clear poverty thresholds and avoid key forms of deprivation (Fouarge and Layte, 2005; Scruggs and Allan, 2006; Brady et al., 2009).

Note, then, that 'generosity' of welfare does not necessarily equate to 'progressive' outcomes – earnings-related benefits can instead help to sustain structural inequalities (Gugushvili and Hirsch, 2014). Some of the most generous replacement rates are to be found in north-western Europe, and can be as high as 100% for some household types for a certain period following unemployment (this is the case in Denmark, for instance) (OECD, 2015; Wang and Van Vliet, 2016). Less generous systems may fail to raise benefit recipients above the poverty line and leave them unable to meet even their basic needs (Scruggs and Allan, 2006; Saltkjel and Malmberg-Heimonen, 2016). Recent research in the UK, for example, has indicated that mainstream benefit levels for single people under 25 are now so low that, for those living away from the family home with no other source of income, the risks of absolute destitution are extremely high even if they are claiming the full range of benefits to which they are entitled (Fitzpatrick et al., 2016).

A key issue here is the uprating of benefit levels over time, which determines whether (or not) they keep pace with inflation and maintain their real value. In many countries, working-age out-of-work benefits are indexed to consumer price levels (this is the case, for example, in Australia, Belgium, the Czech Republic, France, Luxembourg, New Zealand, Norway, Poland, Switzerland and, until recently, the UK), though in some they are adjusted based on trends in pension benefit levels (as in Austria, Finland, Germany, Hungary, Italy and Portugal) or wages (as in Denmark and the Netherlands) (Wang and Van Vliet, 2016). In Estonia, Ireland and Slovakia, no automatic indexation occurs, with adjustments dependent on discrete government measures (Wang and Van Vliet, 2016).

Below-inflation increases followed by a four-year benefit freeze have eroded the real value of most working-age cash transfers in the UK, and are a key driver of forecasted increases in poverty and inequality (Hood and Waters, 2017a). With respect to housing allowances in particular, their relative generosity may be undermined (or enhanced) by the extent to which they track rising (or falling) rent levels. Again in the UK, limits on local housing allowance rates, together with an overall cap on the total benefits that may be received by out-of-work households, have seen a gap open up between actual rent levels, especially in the private market, and the assistance available to low-income families to meet these costs (Fitzpatrick et al., 2017; National Audit Office, 2017). A shortfall between rent allowances and private sector rents is also a major issue in Australia, where the Productivity Commission recently recommended a 15% increase in Commonwealth Rent Assistance and the introduction of indexation rules that ensure allowance levels keep pace with actual rents (Productivity Commission, 2017).

In terms of duration, more generous welfare systems might make social assistance benefits available on a continuing or indefinite basis, or until the need for support ceases. Less generous systems, on the other hand, impose time limits for individual claims or make access dependent on cash-limited pots. The most striking example of low generosity in terms of the welfare entitlement duration was introduced in the US in 1996 under the radical Personal Responsibility Work Opportunity and Reconciliation Act (PRWORA). Since that time, the main federally-funded cash benefit for low-income families with dependent children, Temporary Assistance for Needy Families (TANF), has been subject to a national lifetime limit of five years. Though states are permitted to fund longer coverage for those exceeding the time limit, the vast majority have introduced this 60-month maximum, and some have instituted even shorter maximum periods. Once this period has expired, and regardless of the acuteness of continuing need, the only help available to such families to meet their basic needs is generally food stamps (via the Supplemental Nutrition Assistance Program), unless particular states have used their own funds and discretion to put in place more generous local provision (Paz-Fuchs, 2008; Narain and Ettner, 2017; Schott, 2012). Even food aid is subject to a time limit (of three months during a three-year period) for certain categories of out-of-work, able-bodied adults without dependants (Falk et al., 2014). In sharp contrast, most European benefit systems and a large number of OECD countries place no such time limits on receipt of (non-contributory) cash benefits, so long as claimants continue to meet relevant eligibility criteria and conditions of access, which often involve a means test (Langenbucher, 2015).

In the social housing sphere, too, there are variations between welfare systems in terms of the duration for which assistance can be received. In many northern European countries social tenants enjoy indefinite 'security of tenure', meaning that they can stay in their property as long as they wish and regardless of changes in their income or circumstances, assuming they abide by the terms of their lease agreement, including meeting rental payments (Fitzpatrick and Pawson, 2011). In the US and Canada, in contrast, public housing tenants must, at least in theory, continue to fulfil certain eligibility criteria, including with respect to having an income below specified thresholds, in order to maintain occupancy of their homes. The deployment of income-related social rents in these jurisdictions is, however, generally said to provide sufficient incentive for higher-income tenants to exit the sector of their own accord without the need to evict them (Fitzpatrick and Pawson, 2011). More recently, in Australia, and now in England, some social landlords have implemented a 'fixed-term' tenancy regime, wherein periodic reviews may see tenancies ended if there is evidence that household circumstances have changed with regard to, for example, employment status, income level or size (Fitzpatrick and Pawson, 2014). The extent to which social landlords will actually use these powers to evict households who no longer meet relevant eligibility criteria remains to be seen, but the policy change does indicate a shift in some quarters from seeing social housing as a 'home for life' to seeing its role more as an 'ambulance' service, temporarily available to those in acute need (see Chapter 4; Fitzpatrick and Watts, 2017).

Finally, with regard to in-kind rather than cash transfer benefits, relative levels of generosity may be associated with the quality of the goods or services provided for free or at a reduced (subsidised) cost. For example, the quality of emergency, transitional and longer-term accommodation and support available to homeless people varies considerably across, and within, countries, even just in Europe (Allen, 2012), and so too the building standards, state of repair, energy efficiency and other relevant aspects of social housing (Eurofound, 2016). In education, quality might be operationalised in terms of investment in infrastructure and teacher training, or with reference to outcomes achieved, something increasingly possible to measure, albeit controversial, via the Programme for International Student Assessment (PISA) survey (Meyer and Benavot, 2013). Even with regard to cash benefits, 'quality' may be conceptualised in relation to the accuracy, timeliness and efficiency of the administration of payments: benefit delays have been shown to have important implications for low-income households, including pushing some groups into extreme material deprivation, or destitution, even in advanced welfare economies (Fitzpatrick et al., 2016).

So far we have established that the degree of targeting and relative generosity of cash and in-kind benefits are two quite distinct qualities of welfare systems. Welfare provision may be narrowly targeted at a small group (according to any particular or combination of the status, need and behavioural criteria outlined above), and may at the same time offer generous benefits to those who manage to meet these criteria. This combination may be argued to characterise the welfare settlement in Denmark, for example, which combines stringent active labour market policies and substantial restrictions on benefits owed to recent migrants with unusually high (contributory and social assistance) benefit levels and replacement rates for 'insiders' (Vis et al., 2011; Klein and Hansen, 2016). A very different example can be found in the conditional cash transfer programmes used in developing-country contexts, some of which (the Red de Protección Social program in Nicaragua, for example) combine comparatively generous levels of transfer with narrow targeting at 'extremely poor' households (Fiszbein et al., 2009). Conversely, a focus on relatively widely available but ungenerous out-of-work income maintenance benefits may fairly summarise the pre-2010 UK welfare system (since 2010 UK working-age benefits have become both more highly targeted and even less generous).

More generally, policy makers unwilling or unable to increase investment in welfare provision will face a trade-off between the breadth (degree of targeting) and depth (generosity) of the benefit safety net, which in turn will be determined by ideological preferences, political priorities and/or embedded societal values (Fitzpatrick and Stephens, 2014). It follows that while highly conditional forms of welfare are often assumed to be associated with residual, means-tested and ungenerous welfare policies, this is far from a necessary connection.

## Entitlement

A further important distinction can be drawn between welfare goods and services allocated on the basis of *entitlement* and those distributed according to the *discretion* of local decision makers or service providers.

Welfare entitlements are accessed 'as of right' where the claimant meets the specified criteria and conditions set out in law. In such cases, there is legal obligation, usually on central or local government, or another public body, to satisfy these entitlements, which should be enforceable through relevant courts or tribunals. *Eligibility* and *entitlement* are not synonyms: being eligible for a benefit means that that you *may* receive it, whereas being entitled means that you *must* receive it.

Discretionary forms of welfare, on the other hand, are not a matter of right or entitlement, but are instead distributed according to bureaucratically-defined standards or norms and/or the decision-making of individual officials. According to Goodin (1986), *discretion*

> refers to an area of conduct which is generally governed by rules but where the dictates of rules are indeterminate. In short, discretion refers, negatively, to a lacuna in a system of rules.
>
> *(p.234)*

The basic rationale for discretionary benefits is said to be the need for freedom, flexibility and creativity within welfare systems, particularly with respect to urgent or exceptional needs which may be sudden and unpredictable (Evans, 2016; Hill, 2014). However, another attraction of discretionary programmes for policy makers is the ability to cap expenditure. Whereas entitlement programmes are demand-led, as all who qualify must receive the relevant benefit, discretionary programmes are very often budget-limited, so that many of those who are eligible for benefits may fail to receive them if resources are constrained and need to be rationed (Priemus et al., 2005).

An illuminating contrast can again be drawn here between the UK and US welfare systems (Bambra, 2007). The UK Housing Benefit system, though increasingly conditional and hedged around with restrictions (Stephens and Stephenson, 2016), nonetheless remains entitlement based. Shifts towards increased reliance on locally managed 'Discretionary Housing Payments' to supplement the (ever more restricted) mainstream entitlement benefit remain controversial (Meers, 2014). In the US, on the other hand, the nearest equivalent to Housing Benefit – 'Section 8 Housing Choice Vouchers' – has no entitlement element, and in practice these vouchers are received by only around one quarter of those low-income households eligible for them (US Department of Housing and Urban Development, 2013; Falk et al., 2014).

Discretionary welfare powers do not mean, however, that public officials can act with impunity or make arbitrary decisions. Even where decisions on access to benefits are discretionary, they must nonetheless be lawful, and in the UK are subject to the supervisory jurisdiction of the superior courts (Public Law Project, undated). This means that such decisions are challengeable, at least in theory, by way of judicial review procedures if they are not made in a rational, reasonable and proportional manner, with all relevant considerations, such as official guidance, given due weight and all irrelevant considerations, including personal prejudices, disregarded (Loveland, 1992; see also Robson and Poustie, 1996). Discretion therefore doesn't imply *license*, but rather that officials are able to choose between two or more equally valid courses of action (Goodin, 1986; Walker, 2005).

The concept of discretion was key to Lipsky's (1980/2010) account of the power of 'street-level bureaucrats', that is, public service workers who interact directly with citizens in the course of their jobs. A large literature from Lipsky (1980/2010) onwards has sought to establish that official discretion is inescapable in welfare policy implementation, even in the case of entitlement-based provision, with street-level bureaucrats best understood as 'de facto policy-makers' (Lipsky, 1980/2010, p.24). Relevant authors emphasise that 'discretion is inherent in welfare delivery, even in the most apparently rule-bound system' (Brodkin, 1997, p.4; see also Hill, 2014) and that street-level bureaucrats in job centres, welfare-to-work programmes, municipal housing authorities and so on develop 'adaptive responses' to their organisational environment. These practices, when they become systematic, 'can result in rationing, sorting, selectivity and other common practices that occur beneath the radar of most oversight' (Brodkin, 2013, p.23).

Donnison (1977), however, draws a helpful distinction between *judgement*, that is the interpretation and application of rules (for instance, the decision as to whether a particular individual is in fact sick, disabled or homeless), and *discretion*, which leaves space within a system of rules for officials to make a decision as they see fit. For example, in the case of UK unemployment benefit, bureaucrats must interpret (or *judge* in Donnison's terms) whether a particular claimant is eligible to receive benefits and available for work, but work coaches then have discretion (which has been broadened under Universal Credit) in specifying the precise level of work search requirements to be placed on that individual in their 'Claimant Commitment' (e.g. the number of applications or hours of job search activity required per week, and frequency of appointments at the Jobcentre) and the 'infractions' that will lead to sanction (Cain, 2016). Discretionary powers also exist elsewhere in the system: though the now highly controversial Work Capability Assessments are supposed to ensure consistency, assessors can make use of discretionary 'special circumstances' regulations where they consider someone at substantial risk of harm if found fit for work (Baumberg et al., 2015). Similarly, work coaches can choose to make use of discretionary 'easements', suspending or reducing work search requirements for particular 'special needs' groups, for instance those experiencing homelessness (Batty et al., 2015). In line with Hill's (2014) expectation that bureaucrats will rarely use discretion to 'do significantly more than they could', it appears that such easements are, at least to date, infrequently used (Johnsen et al., 2016; Batty et al., 2015).

According to Donnison (1977), while judgement is inescapable in public bureaucracies, discretion can be reduced (and even eliminated) by rules restricting its scope. A stark example of how policy frameworks can expand or contract the room for discretion (or the 'lacuna in a system of rules') is provided by a comparison of Scotland's legal-rights-based and Ireland's non-rights-based response to homelessness. Focusing on the experiences of single homeless men, Watts (2014) found that the framework of clear legal entitlements owed to virtually all homeless households in Scotland 'crowded out' the discretion of service providers to a very significant degree. In Ireland, in contrast, absent the legally enforceable rehousing duties incumbent on local authorities in Scotland, concerns regarding 'housing readiness', desert, social mix and local reactions to rehousing particular individuals played a substantial role in brokering access to housing for single homeless men, even though these issues were not explicitly articulated in official policy.

Disquiet about discretion in public welfare often reflects the sense that welfare users should not have to rely on the 'goodwill' of public officials to receive benefits that meet their basic needs, and that it can lead to inconsistency, bias and inequity and, at worst, 'petty officials' (Goodin, 1986, p.233) administrating 'semi-charitable hand-outs' (Donnison, 1977, p.534). The association, and sometimes conflation, of discretionary and charitable provision may reflect that beneficiaries of both kinds of assistance can be viewed as passive recipients of largesse; as humiliated supplicants, rather than legitimate and empowered 'rights holders' (Le Grand, 1997; Lister, 2004). For those on the political Left, this can mean that discretionary benefits are also vulnerable to some of the other critiques of 'private charity' (Plant, 1998), i.e. that they are uneven in their coverage, inadequate in what they provide, and ill-targeted at recipients who are most desirable, presentable or articulate, rather than those in most need (Digby, 1989; Singer, 2015; Parsell and Watts, 2017). On the other hand, 'entitlement programmes' are anathema to some on the political Right who place a particular premium on the virtue of self-reliance and reject welfare policies that are viewed as inculcating the highly undesirable internalization of a *sense of* entitlement (a 'something for nothing' 'culture of dependence') that offends certain norms of personal responsibility and reciprocity (Mead, 1986; Murray, 1990, 1994; Dunn, 2014; Perkins, 2016).

For some, particularly on the political Left, the very idea of 'rights' brings to mind a moral entitlement that holds regardless of people's conduct (Dwyer, 2004). But if rights are understood more specifically as individually enforceable legal entitlements to specific goods or services (Fitzpatrick et al., 2014), rather than as abstract and universal 'human rights', there is no immediate tension between welfare provision being rights-based and access being conditional on behaviour (see also Chapter 6). In fact, one could question whether the whole concept of 'welfare conditionality' makes sense outside of a (legal) rights-based framework, given that conditionality implies the structuring of access via rules and procedural requirements, and that a definite outcome follows if relevant requirements are met.

However, in one important sense, behavioural conditionality does appear to blur the boundary between rights-based and discretionary provision. This is because conduct conditions are highly likely to expand the space for official discretion, or at least more frequent subjective judgement calls (Donnison, 1977). Watson (2015), for instance, argues that the role of those administering welfare services is 'altered substantially' in more (behaviourally) conditional systems, and that bureaucrats are 'endowed with higher levels of discretion vis-à-vis their clients than are their counterparts in rights-based [i.e. not behaviourally conditional] systems' (p.648).

Rather than simply using their judgement to decide whether claimants meet 'factual' conditions based on easily identifiable broad categories such as age or legal citizenship status, welfare providers administering behaviourally conditional entitlements must assess whether claimants' conduct has met required standards. This is almost inevitably a subjective process to at least some extent, with a tendency to cast decision makers in the role of policing the 'deservingness' of claimants, something more usually associated with discretionary rather than rights-based approaches.

It should be noted, though, that this issue is not unique to *behavioural* forms of conditionality, with higher levels of judgement and discretion also more likely in the administration of entitlements dependent on individuals meeting particular *needs* thresholds. An obvious example is the assessments of 'vulnerability' that abound across much of health, social care, housing and homelessness policies, and often play a central role in rationing access to all manner of welfare interventions (Brown, 2016; Bretheron et al., 2013). Key here is how specific and easily applied, or amorphous and vague, behavioural and other conditionality requirements are. The nature of these requirements is the matter to which we turn our attention in Chapter 3.

## Concluding comments

Our consideration of the context of conditionality in this chapter has highlighted that behavioural conditionality is only one way in which the design of welfare support structures can vary between different jurisdictions. Other forms of targeting based on people's status or needs also play a crucial role in defining who can and who cannot benefit from welfare services. Furthermore, how generous welfare support is, and whether it is provided on the basis of entitlement or discretion, are other vital variables in understanding the shape and strength of social safety nets.

While in advanced welfare states in particular behavioural conditionality has often come to be associated with 'neo-liberal' and 'austerity' reform agendas, this is not a necessary connection. Indeed, as will be explored in more depth in Chapters 3 and 4, we find that conduct conditionality takes a huge variety of forms, and is found in a diverse range of contexts, from Scandinavian welfare states renowned for their universalism to liberal welfare regimes known for their targeted nature and relative lack of generosity, to developing world contexts where conditional approaches form part of the growth and development of fledgling welfare institutions. Moreover, the policy intentions driving such approaches, and their efficacy and impacts, are also hugely diverse (see Chapters 4 and 5). The complex and divergent ethical dilemmas and challenges that this all poses is the theme taken up again in Chapter 6.

# 3

# THE TECHNIQUES OF CONDITIONALITY

'Conditionality' can be thought of as a first-tier concept, requiring deconstruction into its constituent components to be fully understood (Knotz and Nelson, 2013; Adler and Terum, 2017). We propose that conditional forms of welfare with a conduct component differ from other forms of welfare provision in three key respects: they specify *behavioural requirements* which determine initial access to and/or continued receipt of benefits, goods and services; they employ *monitoring and surveillance processes* that verify compliance with those requirements; and they impose *sanctions* in the event of non-compliance or, in some cases, offer *incentives* for compliance. In this chapter, we provide an anatomy of conditionality by exploring these constituent 'techniques' in greater detail.

## Behavioural requirements

In their consideration of conditional benefit systems, Griggs and Evans (2010) distinguish between *administrative* and *behavioural* conduct conditions, emphasising that receipt of benefits is always dependent upon certain 'actions' associated with the processing of claims and maintenance of entitlement (e.g. responding to letters, attending interviews, giving required information) (see also Spicker, 2005; Paz-Fuchs, 2008; Dwyer, 2010). Nevertheless, the shift towards more robust behaviour-related conditionality noted above is widely considered to mark a significant qualitative shift in the nature of welfare provision (Dwyer, 2010). For Clasen and Clegg (2007), this represents a 'new' form of risk management, founded on a '"new politics of the welfare" ... intent on converting the welfare benefits system into a lever for changing behaviour' (Rodger, 2008, p.87; see also Deacon, 2004; Dwyer, 2004; Paz-Fuchs, 2008). Writing in 2004 in the UK context, Deacon describes

> a broad and far-reaching shift towards greater conditionality in welfare. The idea that those claiming welfare should be required to fulfil conditions regarding their own behaviour and that of their children has been extended across a swathe of social policy; from welfare to work, to education, health, and, of course, housing.
>
> *(Deacon, 2004, pp.911–912)*

Conduct conditionality takes a variety of forms depending on the behaviour it seeks to encourage or deter, and the focus, design and overall societal objectives of the specific welfare intervention in question (Bastagli, 2009). As discussed in Chapter 2, one key distinction is between preconditions which determine *initial access* (retrospective behavioural requirements) and/or ongoing behavioural requirements monitored throughout the welfare claim and which determine *continued access*. The classic example of retrospective behavioural conditionality is the widespread restriction of access to out-of-work benefits in cases where a person's unemployment is deemed 'voluntary' following, for example, resignation without 'good cause' or dismissal due to (mis) conduct. In such cases, access to unemployment benefits is frequently postponed, and in countries as diverse as Canada, Greece, South Korea, the Netherlands, Romania and Turkey such individuals may be unable to claim out-of-work benefits at all (see Langenbucher, 2015). Ongoing behavioural requirements, on the other hand, typically include connecting unemployment benefits to prescribed job search activities and evidencing 'availability for work', but may also involve other compulsory activities such as attending training or skills enhancement courses, committing to personal development programmes or, as is discussed below, even undertaking mandatory work activities.

Amplifying this sort of distinction, Flint (2009b) distinguishes between 'conditional' and 'earned' citizenship, with the former referring to 'pre-existing entitlements being rescinded as a result of inappropriate conduct' (Flint, 2009b, p.89), such as failure to meet job search requirements. 'Earned citizenship', on the other hand, denotes the idea that entitlements must be secured *in the first place* by proactive endeavour. Examples of the latter include the linking of social housing tenancies to employment status or compulsory 'volunteering' duties (Fitzpatrick and Watts, 2017), or tying migrants' welfare entitlements to community contribution or language requirements (Flint, 2009b; Dwyer, 2016). This latter trend, something for which 'social democratic' Denmark is particularly renowned, is sometimes referred to as 'welfare chauvinism' by its critics, but seen as necessary to resolving the 'migration/welfare-state paradox' – referring to a claimed tension between sustaining high levels of immigration and the social cohesion required to support a generous welfare state – by its proponents (Anderson, 2007; Kremer, 2016).

Paz-Fuchs (2008) draws a further distinction between welfare that is conditional on 'amorphous' or vague requirements (such as behaving responsibly), and concrete and tightly specified requirements (such as accepting any job offer). Some behavioural requirements can concern matters as complex and multi-faceted as whether someone made themselves homeless 'intentionally', a question that has generated reams of case law in the UK, where certain homeless households have a legally enforceable right to be rehoused by their local authority as long as they have not brought about their homelessness through their own actions or inaction (Robson and Poustie, 1996; Cowan, 2011). Striking a similar note, new homelessness legislation in Wales, and now in England, requires homeless applicants to 'cooperate' with housing officers' efforts to prevent or relieve their homelessness or else lose their entitlement to be rehoused (Mackie et al., 2017).

Conduct requirements also differ in that they may encapsulate positive requirements to engage in certain behaviour or negative requirements to desist from particular behaviour. Positive requirements can range from work search or work readiness activities to enrolling children in school or attending health-related appointments (see Chapter 4). A particularly controversial 'positive' behavioural requirement is to be found in the style of 'workfare' pioneered from 1997 in Wisconsin in the US, whereby welfare recipients have to 'earn' their benefits via compulsory work programmes. Specific requirements could involve placement in subsidised or unsubsidised employment, unpaid work experience in community service jobs (classic US 'workfare'), or supported work or work-related activities, including, for instance, drug or health treatment, for those with multiple barriers to employment. These compulsory work activities typically take place in charity shops, office or customer service work environments, or in the provision of care or in 'light industrial and housekeeping work' (Crisp and Fletcher, 2008, p.10). Workfare programmes are also common in other Anglosphere countries, such as Australia and Canada, and the Netherlands has a 'Work First' scheme modelled on the Wisconsin programme (Lindsay et al., 2007).

There has been recent controversy in England over short-term Mandatory Work Activity requirements and work experience schemes (Daguerre and Etherington, 2014). Resistance to this form of workfare came from several quarters, not least the Social Security Advisory Committee (an advisory public body), but also from activists and campaigners (for instance the Boycott Workfare campaign). Mandatory Work Activity was also subject to formal legal challenge, with two cases eventually leading to a court ruling that benefit claimants being 'forced to work for free' was illegal. However, the challenge was successful on procedural grounds (linked to the information provided to claimants in the course of implementing workfare), rather than on the basis that participation in unpaid work as a condition of benefit receipt was in and of itself illegal or a form of 'forced labour', as critics had claimed (Hern, 2013). Nevertheless, the controversy fuelled a highly sensitive parallel legal challenge which eventually forced the UK government to release the names of over 500 placement provider organisations (including many charities) who had participated in the scheme (Staufenberg and Stone, 2016).

Negative requirements to cease or refrain from doing something tend to be less common in cash benefits programmes, though not unheard of. In the US, the Personal Responsibility and Work Act 1996 (PRWORA) introduced provisions that permanently denied cash assistance and food stamps to individuals convicted of a drug-related felony, and reduced the entitlements of families that included an individual with such a conviction (Paz-Fuchs, 2008). In 2007, the UK's New Labour government introduced provisions to sanction the housing allowance of families who failed to desist from anti-social behaviour or engage in support to address it, although these were not rolled out following mixed evaluation results from a small-scale pilot (Flint et al., 2011). Requirements that prohibit certain forms of behaviour are more frequently found in the design of in-kind benefits programmes, particularly those related to housing and homelessness, where keeping one's tenancy or a place in supported accommodation unit is generally predicated on refraining from anti-social or disruptive behaviour. In one particularly stark example of such a negative (pre)condition, again from the US, people with drug convictions have in the past faced a lifetime ban from accessing public housing, known as *One Strike and You're Out* policies. Federal provisions excluding this group were strengthened in the 1980s and 1990s, but public housing authorities have more recently been encouraged to soften their approach in line with the 2008 Second Chance Act, which aimed to promote the rehabilitation of offenders and reduce recidivism (Walter et al., 2017).

Behavioural conditions may also vary substantially in how onerous they are, ranging from a simple requirement to 'sign on' as actively seeking work on a regular basis to much more time-intensive job search requirements, all the way through to personally challenging activities such as learning a new language or addressing addiction issues. For instance, the minimum number of 'job search actions' required varies from being unspecified, to being specified but low (two per month in Japan, Korea and Latvia), to as many as 20 per month in metropolitan areas in Australia (Langenbucher, 2015). In the UK, Universal Credit claimants are required to demonstrate active job search activities for up to 35 hours per week (Dwyer and Wright, 2014). In the US, individuals who are out of work and over 18, but have not completed high school, are subject to stringent Individual Responsibility Plans, which can involve requirements to attend school, maintain grades and undergo treatment for any substance misuse issues

(Paz-Fuchs, 2008). In several US states, recipients who have tested positive in drugs tests can only maintain access to benefits (or regain it after a certain period of disqualification) if they comply with substance abuse treatment plans and test negative at the end of treatment (NCSL, 2017). Proposals to reform social security benefits as a lever to force people to address drug or alcohol addictions (e.g. through drug testing), and other health and 'lifestyle' issues like obesity, have also emerged elsewhere in the Anglosphere countries in recent years, including in Canada, the UK and Australia, though in many cases they have not yet progressed into law given their highly controversial reception and concerns about their likely efficacy (Wincup, 2014; Black, 2016; Pérez-Muñoz, 2017).

While requirements are often standard and uniform for all those eligible for the welfare good or service in question, in some cases they may be partially or fully personalised to the targeted individuals' circumstances, needs or capabilities. In the latter case, requirements might be negotiated or 'co-produced' between the individual targeted and the relevant welfare provider, or imposed by professional decision makers. The UK's Jobseekers' 'Claimant Commitments', which specify the work search requirements that unemployed claimants must undertake, are, in theory, developed through dialogue between an employment adviser and claimant, though the extent of this tailoring and co-production in practice has been disputed (Batty et al., 2015).

Friedli and Stearn (2015) argue that so-called 'psychological conditionality' is also increasingly evident in UK social security programmes. By this they mean conditions which require those who are out of work not simply to *behave* in particular ways (i.e. turn up to appointments and/or apply for a certain number of jobs every week) but also 'to demonstrate certain *attitudes or attributes*' [emphasis added], namely 'work-appropriate' and positive attitudes, beliefs and dispositions including confidence, assertiveness, optimism and aspiration (p.40). Friedli and Stearn share personal testimony from people who have been threatened with a sanction for not participating adequately in team work or role-play exercises due to shyness; who have been criticised by work coaches for having the 'wrong attitude' to work search; and who have been referred by welfare-to-work providers to mandatory psychological evaluations. This 'psycho-compulsion' they argue represents 'the recruitment of psychology – and, by implication, psychologists – into monitoring, modifying and punishing people who claim social security benefits' (Friedli and Stearn, 2015, p.42) and reflects an understanding of unemployment as a 'psychological failure' (p.45) rather than in relation to wider socio-economic trends.

## Monitoring and verification

Conditional forms of welfare necessarily rely on processes of monitoring and verification to assess whether the relevant behavioural requirements have been met. Effective claimant supervision and surveillance is core to the logic of conditionality, underpinning as it does the credibility of the threat of sanction that is key to this particular 'coercive' method of bringing about behavioural change (Raja, 2014; Bastagli, 2009; Fiszbein et al., 2009; McVicar, 2010). Monitoring and verification processes vary substantially on a number of dimensions, particularly with respect to what precisely is monitored, who undertakes this process and when and how they do so.

Exactly *what* is being monitored can range from overt and easily observable behaviour or actions (e.g. attendance at an appointment); to more subjective measures of engagement, commitment, performance or improvement in various tasks; to much-harder-to-observe attitudinal or dispositional considerations (see above). This also means that what is being monitored may vary in terms of how directly or indirectly it tracks the behavioural responses sought by the policy. We can illustrate via the example of 'Conditional Cash Transfers' (CCTs) often used in developing-world contexts to increase low-income families' take-up of health care and education services (see Chapter 4 for details). In some cases, such as requirements around child immunisation or school enrolment, monitoring the *actual behaviour* sought may be possible via medical and school records, depending on the capacity, skills and infrastructure of those institutions. In other schemes, it is the *desired outcome* – children's performance at school – that is monitored and linked to CCTs. Where the intended behaviour or behavioural outcome is harder to measure directly – for example, more nutritious eating, effective budgeting or better parenting practice – proxy measures such as attendance at classes aiming to develop these skills may be used (Fiszbein et al., 2009; Pellerano and Barca, 2014). A key question in the design and effectiveness of conditional welfare is therefore how desired behaviours are translated into explicit requirements that can be effectively monitored (Pellerano and Barca, 2014).

Consequently, *how* compliance is measured and verified can also vary substantially. To use the example of unemployment benefits this time, claimants are often asked to self-report their compliance. However, what this means in practice can vary from simply ticking a box to confirm that they have been actively seeking work to providing a detailed account of their work search activities including evidence or documentation such as a diary or log of actions undertaken. These logs may have to include specific details of jobs applied for, contact details of the employer (for decision makers to verify or spot check) and even – as is the case in Malta – a declaration from prospective employers that an application or enquiry has been made (Langenbucher, 2015). Alternatively, monitoring may be separated from claimants' recording of it, for instance, with job search required to take place via a particular website or app which can be directly monitored by officials (the Universal Job Match website serves this purpose in the UK). In some rare cases, assessment of compliance and associated sanctions is automated. In New York City, for instance, computer systems are programmed to initiate sanctions where they register that a client has not attended required work activity (Lens, 2008; Raja, 2014).

These examples also serve to illustrate the sheer breadth of actors who may be involved in monitoring and verification, including the claimant, the organisation providing the service or access to the benefit (local or national government or a commissioned external service) and a range of potential intermediary actors, including the employers to which out-of-work benefit claimants apply for jobs, or the employability, health care or education providers that claimants may be mandated to engage with (Fiszbein et al., 2009). In Sweden and Norway social assistance programmes are professionalised and staffed by social workers afforded high levels of discretion, whereas in the US they are bureaucratic organisations staffed by non-professionals more likely to be subject to strict regulation, targets and performance-management processes (Jewell, 2007; Terum et al., 2017).

Given that assessment of compliance is rarely an automated process, but rather one involving multiple human actors, it is possible that discriminatory attitudes and prejudice influence these processes. Two studies undertaken in the US and Norway employed vignettes in surveys of welfare caseworkers to measure the extent and nature of discriminatory practice in the implementation of activation programmes. Schram et al. (2009) found that in the US, case workers were more likely to sanction claimants with Spanish- or African American-sounding names than those with Caucasian names if the claimant violated programme requirements. In a recent Norwegian study of 1,700 frontline workers, by contrast, Terum et al. (2017) found evidence of *reverse* discrimination: those with a North African name were less frequently sanctioned that those with a native Norwegian name. The authors argue that this stark difference likely reflects the contrasting level of professionalisation of social assistance programmes mentioned above, as well as broader institutional-cultural contextual differences.

Many programmes including a conditional element include an appeals process: this is the case, for instance, in relation to the UK's benefit sanction regime, sanctions associated with the Temporary Assistance for Needy Families Programme (TANF) in the US, and in Sweden, where sanctions associated with activation programmes can be appealed in administrative courts. Controversy, however, has surrounded appeals processes, with concern in the UK, for instance, that claimants face considerable disincentives in appealing sanctions decisions given the onerous and lengthy nature of relevant processes, during which they will be suffering the effects of the sanction (Webster, 2015a; Adler, 2016; Adler and Terum, 2017). There have been a number of attempts to challenge the fundamental idea that behavioural conditions can be attached to unemployment benefits via the European Court of Human Rights, though none have been successful thus far (Adler and Terum, 2017).

Finally, *when* compliance is monitored and verified will also vary, ranging from intermittently (for instance, yearly verification of school enrolment in the case of CCTs to families) to more regularly (monthly, fortnightly, weekly or daily attendance at appointments or training sessions). In some countries (Denmark, Bulgaria, Finland, Germany,

Ireland, New Zealand, Slovak Republic, and Slovenia) work search efforts usually need to be demonstrated quarterly, or less frequently. In others (Australia, Portugal and the UK), they must be demonstrated fortnightly, and in some instances even more often (Langenbucher, 2015). In the UK, some groups of the long-term unemployed can be placed on a 'daily work search regime' (Dar, 2016).

Frequent 'surveillance' is also a core element of Family Intervention Projects, used in the UK to address anti-social behaviour and support 'troubled' families with multiple problems (Flint, 2009a, 2012). Within such programmes home visits by support workers – sometimes daily – are a core element of the support which must be accepted to retain an 'under threat' social housing tenancy. In some cases surveillance may be more or less continuous; for instance, in the case of 24-hour supported residential homelessness services with behavioural requirements around anti-social behaviour, alcohol or drug consumption or engagement with support plans (Parsell, 2016). While commentary on such intensive monitoring and surveillance in welfare provision has tended to focus on its intrusive and disciplinary nature, several contributions to these debates have highlighted that such surveillance can also be experienced as supportive and inclusive, by enabling tailored support (Flint, 2009a, 2012), and in the case of vulnerable individuals living in congregate supportive housing programmes, conducive to feelings of safety (Parsell, 2016).

Monitoring and verification processes are therefore an indispensable feature of conditional programmes, but come with a financial cost in terms of infrastructure and staff time (Bastagli, 2009; Fiszbein et al., 2009), albeit that these will vary depending on the intensity, frequency and extent of the surveillance undertaken. There are also costs to claimants or recipients, both in terms of time spent demonstrating compliance, and also sometimes in financial terms (see Chapter 5). There are other, less tangible, costs too, with higher levels of 'judgment and intrusion into a client's personal life' required to assess whether claimants meet behavioural requirements than those required to assess other kinds of eligibility criteria or thresholds of need (Watson, 2015, p.648; see also Flint, 2006; Flint and Nixon, 2006; Pérez-Muñoz, 2017). The ethical dilemmas and trade-offs these issues pose are explored in Chapter 6.

## Sanctions

Perhaps the most distinctive element of behaviourally-conditional forms of welfare is the sanction itself, that is, the loss or deprivation imposed on the recipient or claimant as a consequence of failure to complying with the conduct requirements. It is this 'punitive' aspect of conditionality that attracts most controversy, and some have drawn parallels with criminal justice policy, wherein sanctions such as fines or imprisonment are used to achieve policy goals of deterrence, retribution and/or restitution (Fletcher, 2013; Fletcher and Wright, 2017). Webster (2015a), for instance, has likened the highly conditional aspects of the British benefit system to a 'secret penal system', exacting harsh penalties on a very high volume of 'wrongdoers', while lacking the safeguards of transparency and accountability associated with the mainstream judicial system (see also Adler, 2016).

Intensified welfare conditionality has more generally been understood in relation to trends towards what Loic Waquant describes in a visually striking metaphor as 'the centaur state':

> liberal at the top and paternalistic at the bottom ... [presenting] radically different faces at the two ends of the social hierarchy: a comely and caring visage toward the middle and upper classes, and a fearsome and frowning mug towards the lower class.
>
> *(Wacquant, 2009, p.312)*

Central to this characterisation is the increased use of sanctions, both criminal (manifest in burgeoning prison populations in many developed welfare states, particularly the US but also in the UK) and, crucially, via the welfare state (Fletcher, 2013; Flint, forthcoming), with respect to low-income populations, while much milder 'nudge'-type interventions are typically employed to steer better-off groups towards desired patterns of behaviour (see further in Chapter 5).

The concept of sanctions has received considerable attention in political, legal and social theory, and in the late eighteenth century Jeremy Bentham (1791/1995; see also Hirschi and Gottfredson, 2005; Chriss, 2007; Jacques and Allen, 2013) distinguished between five types of sanction, based on the *source* from which the relevant 'pain' flows:

- *Political* or *legal* sanctions are dispensed by government officials for violations of administrative, criminal or civil law, and take the form, for instance, of imprisonment or fines;
- *Sympathetic* sanctions refer to grief arising from someone's own conscience;
- *Moral* or *social* sanctions are meted out by community members/ other human beings, such as exclusion from a social group or an expression of disappointment; historically, and in certain contexts today, such sanctions also include violence (Pinker, 2011);
- *Religious* sanctions are the product of supernatural power, primarily conceived of as received upon death, but also prefigured by moral or social sanctions within the relevant religious community or dispensed by religious 'authorities';
- *Physical* or *natural* sanctions result from natural processes/interacting with the natural environment.

One way of reframing this typology is in terms of the 'distance' between the behaviour in question and the sanction. At one extreme, physical sanctions are (often) certain and (tend to be) immediate (e.g. being burned by a flame); at the other extreme, political or legal sanctions are 'notoriously uncertain and much delayed' (Hirschi and Gottfredson, 2005, p.217), and supernatural sanctions are an article of faith.

Chriss (2007) discusses sanctions, in the context of his broader analysis of social control, as a mechanism via which '*members of society attempt to assure the norm-conforming behaviour of others*' (p.12). He makes two key distinctions. The first (which overlays with Bentham's typology) distinguishes between centralised sanctions – meted out by formal agents of a centralised state, e.g. via the courts of law – and diffuse sanctions – meted out on a face-to-face, informal basis by small groups or communities. The second distinction focuses on who the target of the sanction is: individual sanctions apply to the person who violated the norm/rule in question, whereas collective sanctions target a group as a result of the actions of an individual or several individuals within that group, and as such have long raised particular moral concerns as denoting 'collective punishment'.

Sanctions associated with welfare conditionality might primarily be thought of as 'political/legal' or 'centralised' in that they tend to be defined at the level of national policy (some exceptions are discussed in Chapter 4). However, sanctions are in most cases implemented by 'street-level bureaucrats' (Lipsky, 1980/2010), with greater or lesser amounts of discretion and latitude in how they are interpreted and applied, as discussed above. In practice, then, they are likely to span the 'diffuse' and 'moral/social' categories of Chriss and Bentham, with formal policy mechanisms intermingling with the effects of face-to-face interaction with welfare workers. In addition to formal conditionality and sanctions policies, these workers will have at their disposal (consciously, or not) a range of informal mechanisms of 'moral' and 'social' sanctions that characterise human interaction, i.e. blame, disappointment, stigma, etc. Welfare conditionality might also in practice have effects associated with 'sympathetic sanctions' if, for instance, an emphasis on conduct conditionality leads to internalisation of social stigma by those in receipt of welfare support (Spicker, 1984; Link and Phelan, 2001; Lister, 2004).

Similarly, in relation to Chriss' second distinction between individual and collective sanctions, those associated with welfare conditionality might tend to be thought of as 'individual', in that they target the recipient or claimant of a particular good or service. In reality, however, their practical reach may extend much further. First, welfare sanctions may explicitly target a whole household unit, as can be the case in evictions from social housing – anti-social behaviour may involve only one, or some, members of a family but all can lose their home. Second, even where ostensibly only an individual is the target of a particular sanction, reductions or cessation of benefits can have fairly direct (if unintended) impacts on other household members, dependants and perhaps also on wider networks of family, friends and community. The impact of welfare sanctions of innocent 'third parties' is of particular concern with regard to the children of those who fail to satisfy conduct conditions (Deacon, 2004). The association between the imposition of benefit sanctions and absolute destitution, which has seen large numbers of low-income households unable to afford food and other basic necessities, has been a source of major controversy in the UK (Fitzpatrick et al., 2016; Garthwaite, 2016; Lambie-Mumford, 2017). Welfare sanctions may also, over the longer term, have substantial community impacts, with associated increases in poverty linked, in extremis, to higher rates of child abuse, domestic violence, acquisitive crime and sex work (see Chapter 5).

Beyond these broad typologies, finer-grained distinctions can also be drawn between different kinds of sanction, in particular according to the nature of the 'deprivation' that the sanction imposes. In criminology, a key distinction is drawn between *monetary* and *non-monetary* sanctions (e.g. fines versus imprisonment) (O'Malley, 2009). In social policy, sanctions will very often be monetary, involving the removal or suspension of cash transfers. In other cases, particularly with respect to in-kind programmes of welfare, sanctions may be non-monetary, but nonetheless material, involving exclusion from a particular place, space or facility (e.g. a house, homeless accommodation unit or a day centre) or service (for instance, personal support of some kind).

However, there are sanctions which may not be material at all, but rather take the form of deprivation of freedom or choice. This includes, for instance, 'income management' schemes that restrict how benefit income can be spent, controversially introduced in Australia in such a way as to disproportionately affect Aboriginal communities, and civil orders banning rough sleepers or street drinkers from a particular area, again sometimes highly sensitive interventions as they may be viewed as (unfairly) targeting vulnerable groups (see Chapter 4). Other non-monetary sanctions, such as the use of vouchers or prepaid store cards rather than cash for 'failed' or 'refused' asylum seekers, or as a 'warning system' for those who fail to adhere to work search requirements, can be viewed as making explicit use of non-material sanctions, specifically social stigma, as a means to compel norm-conforming behaviours, with attendant potential impacts on self-esteem, personal dignity and sense of self-worth (see Chapter 6). In some cases, the 'sanction' for non-compliance can take the form of higher levels of compulsory support for the individual in question to help address barriers to compliance. This is the case in some CCT programmes in the Global South (see Bastagli, 2009; Fiszbein et al., 2009; and Chapter 4). Whether such 'support-based sanctions' are experienced as a sanction in the Benthamite sense of involving some experience of 'pain', or more positively, will depend on the nature of that support and the perspective of the person who receives it.

Sanctions can be *threatened*, *imposed* or both, and the impacts of threats or impositions of sanctions may differ (Wu et al., 2006). Indeed, it is the behavioural effects of the *threat* of sanctions that is perhaps of central interest in understanding the effectiveness of conditional welfare as a behaviour change intervention, in the sense that the imposition of a sanction reflects that the 'choice architecture' provided by conditional forms of provision has failed to achieve its desired effect. Griggs and Evans (2010) thus distinguish between '*ex ante*' or anticipatory sanction effects that result from the threat of sanction, and '*ex post*' effects which result from sanctions being imposed. They also highlight that the presence of sanctions within a welfare programme may impact on people's likelihood of taking up the benefit in the first place ('take-up effects'; see Chapter 5). Other relevant factors are the *certainty* of a sanction, that is, the likelihood of a sanction following non-compliant behaviour, and the *accuracy* of sanctions, that is, how often a sanction will be applied erroneously, in the absence of non-compliant behaviour. Raja (2014), for instance, argues that the *credibility* of a threat of sanction – the likelihood that a sanction will result from non-compliance – is fundamental to understanding the effectiveness of conditionality, and yet is a substantial gap in the evidence base on the impacts of conditionality. On the other hand, there is ample evidence regarding the inaccuracy of sanctioning procedures – i.e. the erroneous application of a sanction. In the UK in 2013, for instance, claimants sought a review of a sanction decision in almost a third of all cases, with almost a third of those reviews ending in the claimant's benefit being reinstated (Adler, 2016).

Sanctions also vary in relation to their magnitude, timing and duration (Wu et al., 2006). For instance, benefit sanctions in the case of non-compliance with work search requirements might lower the amount received by a small or large degree, or payments may cease entirely. The reduction/removal of payments may last for anything from a few days to several years or may involve permanent expulsion from access to support (Watts et al., 2014; Langenbucher, 2015). In Sweden, a first sanction amounts to the equivalent of five days' benefit, while in New Zealand refusing a suitable job offer incurs a 13-week benefit suspension. In Denmark, Estonia and Finland benefit payments are suspended indefinitely for this 'first offence', but can be restarted following re-entry into and re-exit from employment (Langenbucher, 2015). In the UK, sanctions can now last up to three years in the most severe cases, but the harshest sanctions pertain in some US states where families can be permanently excluded from benefits (Falk et al., 2014). In 2010, four states reportedly employed such 'lifetime full-family sanctions', with other states frequently employing full-family sanctions of a year (Casey, 2010).

Finally, sanctions may follow immediately after non-compliant behaviour, be delayed or occur after a series of warnings. In Sweden, for instance, first failures to attend the Public Employment Service in Sweden prompt a warning (Langenbucher, 2015), and warning letters giving claimants an opportunity to provide evidence demonstrating a good reason for not meeting requirements have been trialled in the UK following controversy about the fairness of sanction decisions and their impacts (Department for Work and Pensions, 2016). Delays in the imposition of a sanction are often the result of administrative processes, and risk compromising the behavioural impacts of conditionality in that they limit claimants' perception of cause (an 'infraction' of requirements) and effect (sanction) (Griggs and Evans, 2010).

## Incentives

Welfare conditionality can also involve promised access to some kind of a reward as an incentive to comply. This is often how CCTs work in the Global South, in that families who adhere to behavioural requirements, which are usually concerned with matters such as encouraging child attendance at school or parental engagement with health services, receive a cash transfer, as opposed to those who fail to adhere to these behavioural requirements ceasing to receive a cash transfer (Fiszbein et al., 2009). Where social protection systems are less well developed than in advanced welfare states, such incentives are likely to have more to offer as a policy tool than sanctions used against recipients of existing welfare support, given that people will often have very few benefits that can be taken from them.

Some would argue that any attempt to draw a distinction between sanctions and incentives is misguided, as they are in reality 'technically substitutable' equivalents, two sides of the same coin or the mirror image of each other (Schneider and Ingram, 1990, p.516). A sanction can thus be understood as a 'negative incentive', or an incentive understood as a 'positive sanction'. According to Baldwin (1971), for instance, positive sanctions can be 'actual or promised rewards' and negative sanctions 'actual or threatened punishments' (p.21; see also Chriss, 2007). From this perspective, 'penalties and incentives cannot be clearly distinguished' (Brigham and Brown, 1980, p.9). Responding to the motivational prompt represented by both (the threat of) sanctions and the (promise of) rewards leaves the person in a more advantageous position than failing to do so and, economists would argue, ignoring such prompts generates an 'opportunity cost' in the sense of benefits foregone (Baldwin, 1971). Moreover, the sanctions typologies outlined above can all equally be applied to incentives, only in reverse: examples of political, sympathetic, moral, religious and physical incentives spring easily to mind.

An interesting twist on this perspective is offered by Grant, who proposes a definition of incentives that reflects their origin in psychology (as motivators in the absence of an automatic instinct) and in industry (as motivators when market forces fail to motivate in particular directions). *Incentives* refer to an

> extrinsic benefit or a bonus that is neither the natural or automatic consequence of an action nor **a deserved reward or compensation**; a discrete prompt expected to elicit a particular response; and an offer intentionally designed to alter the status quo by motivating a person to choose differently than he or she would be likely to choose in its absence
> *(Grant, 2012, p.43). [emphasis added]*

If incentives and sanctions can be seen as twinned or mirroring concepts, then sanctions too can be understood as fundamentally about motivation, rather than punishment, reward or fairness. Whereas rewards or punishments are seen as merited or deserved, incentives and sanctions simply seek to prompt a specific action or kind of behaviour. The success of an incentive or sanction then can be judged on the basis of whether the behavioural goal sought is achieved efficiently (see Chapter 6).

There might, however, be reasons to resist this line of argument that holds to the fungibility of sanctions and incentives or rewards. For one thing, some may view incentives as inherently more ethical than sanctions because they offer something 'additional' to welfare recipients rather than taking something away from a group who are, by and large, already poor and disadvantaged. Indeed, in Chapter 1 we conceptualised conditionality as a coercive attempt to change behaviour via the 'threat of deprivation', and this approach suggests a fundamental difference with the use of incentives. Grant (2012), however, cautions against assuming that incentives are the benign companion to dastardly sanctions, arguing that incentives are best understood as a mode of manipulative power that can be coercive, and have many unintended, and negative, consequences, including 'crowding out' intrinsic motivations to behave in 'pro-social' ways (see Chapter 6).

But there are other differences between sanctions and incentives that are also in the frame. First, there is the technicality that while sanctions have 'a limit of total deprivation' (aside from cases where an actor is able to impose and enforce a debt) – that is 'A cannot deprive B of what he does not have' (Baldwin, 1971, p.35) – incentives have no equivalent upper limit (in principle).

Second, and of particular significance, is that sanctions and incentives elicit different behavioural responses. Highly influential research in behavioural economics has established that people weigh benefits and losses differently, and are far more concerned to avoid losses than to receive equivalent gains (Kahneman and Tversky, 1979). Such 'loss aversion' suggests that sanctions may – other things being equal – be more impactful than incentives, and there is some evidence to this effect in the context of active labour market policies (Jensen et al., 2003) and in health (Dolan et al., 2012, p.267), though there is contrary evidence in other fields (Jochelson, 2007) (see also Chapter 5). A striking example is offered by research into the use of incentives and sanctions in the treatment of obesity. Financial incentives are often used in schemes to encourage behaviour change among obese patients, but a review of trials in this area found that these have no significant long-term effect on weight loss or its maintenance (Paul-Ebhohimhen and Avenell, 2008). Promising (though not definitive) results, however, were achieved by an alternative approach pursued in one trial, which instead asked participants to pay money into an account, which was returned to them (with a 'bonus') if and only if weight-related targets were met (Dolan et al., 2012). This is a practical policy example of what is sometimes called a 'throffer' (threat plus offer), i.e. an approach combining incentives (the bonus) and sanctions (the loss of 'savings') (Steiner, 1975).

Third, it has been argued that policy-makers are willing to use incentives and sanctions in different circumstances. In particular, the more important the policy goal, the more likely the reliance on sanctions rather than incentives (Handberg, 1980), which makes sense given the potentially more 'effective' nature of sanctions than incentives (see above). The use of incentives has also been argued to reflect a more positive view of human nature (and indeed society at large; see Chapter 1), with those policy-makers who use sanctions more likely to view people as 'basically lazy, [and] wishing to avoid responsibility' (Baldwin, 1971, p.34). It has also been postulated that sanctions may be preferred to incentives for 'aesthetic', presentational or political reasons, in that they are associated with 'courage, honor, and masculinity' and incentives with being 'soft, weak, or lacking in toughness' (Baldwin, 1971, p.34).

Fourth, a somewhat related point is that, as Schneider and Ingram (1990) suggest, 'Whether a target population's behavior is controlled through positive or negative devices may have more to do with the political power and social status of the target population than with the behavior' (p.517). This accords with the observed asymmetry of welfare conditionality, in that while the middle classes in the UK and elsewhere benefit substantially from public welfare (in the form of tax relief, allowances and the subsidised benefits of employment; see Titmuss, 1958; Dwyer, 2010), they rarely face the kinds of conditions on its receipt that poorer households reliant on out-of-work benefits or other forms of social welfare are subject to (Dwyer, 1998; Flint, 2002; Deacon, 2004; Standing, 2011). While in some other areas of public policy it has been argued that sanctions are harder to portray as legitimate than incentives (Baldwin, 1971), this does not appear to read across to the welfare sphere, where the 'othering' of benefit recipients may rather act to bolster public support for sanctions-backed conditional reforms (Lister, 2004).

Fifth, and linked with this, is the evidence on potential 'spill-over' and 'scarring' effects of sanctions discussed in Chapter 5. Whereas incentives have been argued to promote self-efficacy – that is 'the conviction that one can successfully execute the behaviour required to produce the outcomes [sought]' (Bandura, 1977, cited in Darnton, 2008, p.13) – sanctions risk prompting or reinforcing feelings of personal failure (Jochelson, 2007; Darnton, 2008). The potential greater efficacy of sanctions suggested by 'loss aversion' (see above) must thus be weighed against these costs.

## Concluding comments

Our consideration of the techniques of conditionality in this chapter has highlighted the enormous diversity captured under the banner of welfare conditionality. Though conditional approaches share a core logic – involving the imposition of behavioural requirements, monitoring and verification, and the use of sanctions (or sometimes incentives) – real-world examples reveal wide variations in the design and specification of these components in practice. In some cases welfare conditionality refers to programmes with very stringent or challenging behavioural requirements (e.g. 35 hours a week job search activity, learning a new language, overcoming an addiction), harsh sanctions (e.g. permanent 'full-family' sanctions in parts of the US, up to three years without benefits in the UK), and quite intrusive levels of surveillance (e.g. compulsory daily visits by a support worker). But in many cases the conduct requirements are much more modest, the sanctions relatively mild, or actually incentive-based, and the support offered experienced as reassuring or protective. These differences are likely to correspond to divergent impacts on the ground, and thus to raise very different questions regarding the ethics and justifiability of conditional approaches. Before turning to these matters in Chapters 5 and 6 respectively, the next chapter considers how these diverse modes of welfare conditionality play out in their application to specific groups frequently targeted by these interventions.

# 4

# THE SUBJECTS OF CONDITIONALITY

This chapter focuses on the subjects of behavioural conditionality, that is, groups of welfare recipients who have been targeted by conduct conditions seeking to ensure that they behave (or cease to behave) in particular kinds of ways. A range of examples of conduct conditionality from across the advanced welfare democracies, and also from the Global South, are examined in order to explore the continuities and discontinuities in the rationales for targeting conditionality at these groups, the specific mechanisms employed, and ways these have evolved over time.

We begin by focusing on the 'classic' group targeted by behavioural conditionality – **unemployed people** – who are typically subject to work-related forms of conditionality within the benefit system. We pay specific attention to the targeting of **young people** and **sick and disabled people** within these labour-market-orientated conditional welfare programmes. We then move on to consider the sometimes very different rationales for conditional forms of welfare targeting **low-income families with children**, wherein behaviour change is sought primarily in the education, health and child protection spheres. Finally, we consider conditional forms of welfare in the housing realm, specifically those targeted on **social tenants** and **homeless people**.

## Unemployed people

In its archetypal form, the central objective of welfare conditionality is to (re)integrate unemployed people back into the labour market. Moral narratives about a dependent 'underclass' have been particularly influential in English-speaking countries (especially the US, but also the UK), while 'activation' narratives have been more influential in Continental Europe. Together, these ideas have informed the appeal of conditional approaches to out-of-work benefits across a wide range of developed economies and amongst governments across the political spectrum. We consider both of these overarching narratives, and their policy impacts, before focusing on the specific targeting of young people and sick and disabled people within work-orientated welfare conditionality.

### *Tackling an underclass? The Anglosphere debate*

The idea (if not the explicit language) of an 'underclass' existing at the 'bottom' of society has a long history; in the UK this spans at least back to the sixteenth-century Poor Laws. Beyond the UK, it has been linked to the Marxist distinction between the proletariat and lumpenproletariat, with the latter said to be 'a recruiting ground for thieves and criminals of all sorts' (Marx, 1851, quoted in Welshman, 2013, p.20). From as far back as the 1880s there has been concern about a 'social residuum', following through into recurring twentieth-century 'moral panics' about 'the unemployable', 'problem families', 'the culture of poverty' and 'the cycle of deprivation'. The discursive ground was therefore well laid for the arrival of the incendiary underclass concept into the public and political imagination in the 1980s (Welshman, 2013).

The underclass concept captures notions of a group both *dependent* and *delinquent* (Dean and Taylor-Gooby, 1992), which is 'structurally separate and culturally distinct from traditional patterns of "decent" working class life' (MacDonald, 1997, p.1). Drawing on the characterisation of members of this social strata as lacking a work ethic, being involved in crime and exhibiting high rates of single motherhood, Bagguley and Mann (1992) coined the pithy and memorable phrase 'idle thieving bastards' as shorthand for the depiction of this group by proponents of the underclass thesis. In the US, the theme of racially segregated inner-city ghettos was also central to the notion of an underclass (whose members could then be castigated by those so minded as 'idle thieving Black bastards'?).

Pivotal to popularising the underclass concept was the thinking of US conservative commentator Charles Murray, whose 1984 book *Losing Ground* offered a radical analysis of American social policy since 1950. Murray saw welfare support as harming the very communities it was designed to help by creating incentives for poor people to disengage from work and have children out of wedlock. This analysis formed the basis of his prescription that all state-guaranteed cash benefits (besides short-term unemployment insurance schemes) should be withdrawn, including (specifically) support to single mothers. By enforcing economic self-reliance on groups dependent on welfare, such a move would, in Murray's view, regenerate work norms, enhance personal responsibility and bolster family authority. Murray visited a number of deprived areas in the UK (Birkenhead in Liverpool and Easterhouse in Glasgow) in 1989, reaching the conclusion that Britain too had a growing underclass, albeit smaller, more hidden and less violent than in the US (Murray, 1996). Publicised by the *Sunday Times* and Institute for Economic Affairs, Murray's ideas were extremely influential in the UK, not least in their appeal to the then Prime Minister Margaret Thatcher (Paz-Fuchs, 2008), but also amongst some academics (Dennis, 1993; Dennis and Erdos, 1992).

Coming from a very different perspective, the sociologist William Julius Wilson, in his 1987 book *The Truly Disadvantaged*, offered an account of the underclass that combined structural and cultural factors in explaining the rise of concentrated poverty in American inner cities. He too criticised liberal perspectives that refused to countenance that there are behavioural aspects to these trends, acknowledging that the problems of 'ghetto neighbourhoods' included crime, family dissolution, welfare dependence and low levels of social organisation. However, Wilson's central contention was that these negative behaviours were cultural adaptations to an economic context that severely limited the licit opportunities open to members of the urban underclass. His policy prescriptions therefore focused on programmes to increase employment opportunities (see in particular in his 1997 book *When Work Disappears*).

Writing in a British context, the sociologist (and later lord) Ralf Dahrendorf (1987) also depicted the causes of the underclass in economic terms, emphasising the role of jobless economic growth and labour market deregulation. In his book *Losing Out* (1989), Labour MP Frank Field identified what he viewed as four 'forces of expulsion' driving the emerging UK underclass: unemployment, widening class differences, the exclusion of the very poorest from rapidly rising living standards, and a hardening of public attitudes. Field did not subscribe to the view that this underclass shared a set of deviant attitudes (Lister, 1996), but instead described the exclusion of these groups in terms of 'the loss of a comprehensive approach to citizenship'.

These impassioned 1980s debates led to neither the renewed comprehensive citizenship called for by Wilson, Field and Dahrendorf, nor to Murray's advocated radical cutback in welfare support. As Lawrence Mead, another conservative American political scientist, noted in his 1986 book *Beyond Entitlement*, 'simply to cut back welfare as ... Murray advise[s], while it would force independence on the recipients, lacks the political support to be carried very far' (p.4). Mead argued that the problem with the welfare state was not, in any case, its size but what he viewed as its 'permissiveness':

> The challenge to welfare statesmanship [*sic*] is not so much to change the extent of benefits as to couple them with serious work and other obligations that would encourage functioning and thus promote the integration of recipients.
>
> *(pp.3–4)*

The mid 1990s saw legislation realising Mead's vision to at least some extent in the US and UK, Canada and Australia (Crisp and Fletcher, 2008). In the US, the Democratic President Bill Clinton signed the Personal Responsibility and Work Opportunities Reconciliation Act (PRWORA) into law in 1996 in the context of running for re-election on the promise to 'end welfare as we know it'. PRWORA established the Temporary Assistance for Needy Families (TANF) programme, limiting receipt of cash assistance to five years over a lifetime, with assistance for 'work-eligible' TANF recipients (mainly single mothers) conditional on engagement with work or training-related activities, albeit that federal legislation allowed states flexibility regarding how these participation standards were fulfilled (Daguerre, 2008; Rector, 2012). PRWORA also introduced provision to permanently disentitle individuals convicted for drugs offences from both cash assistance and food stamps, reflecting not a (future-orientated) behaviour change agenda, but rather a commitment to ensuring moral accountability for past actions (Paz-Fuchs, 2008).

Successive post-1979 Conservative governments ratcheted up behavioural conditionality within the UK benefit system, with a series of social security reviews culminating in the introduction of a 'stricter benefit regime' from the late 1980s, and then Jobseeker's Allowance (JSA) in 1996, a pivotal change which intensified monitoring of unemployed claimants' job-seeking behaviour (see Stewart and Wright, 2014; Watts et al., 2014). The 'New Labour' government elected in 1997 continued in this vein, establishing 'a new contract for welfare' and increased scrutiny of unemployed claimants' job search activities, backed by benefit sanctions in cases of non-compliance. A spike in sanctioning in 2007/08 has been linked to a policy imperative to strengthen behavioural conditionality at that time, under the then Secretary of State John Hutton. In parallel, though, the actively redistributive policies of these New Labour administrations, achieved through Chancellor Gordon Brown's 'tax credit' schemes as well as the social security system, saw major reductions in both pensioner and child poverty between 1997 and 2010, albeit that working-age poverty increased over this period (Hills, 2013).

On coming to power in 2010, the Conservative-led Coalition government pushed forward with a radical programme of welfare cuts including, to date, a freeze in working-age benefit levels, major reductions in housing allowances (affecting younger people in particular), tightened eligibility and reduced generosity in sickness and disability benefits, a 'two-child' limit on child-related benefits and other restrictions in family benefits, and an overall cap on household benefits (affecting larger families in particular) (see Hills, 2014). Fiscally neutral, once parallel tax cuts are taken into account (De Agostini et al., 2014), and disproportionately impacting on the poorest parts of the country

(Beatty and Fothergill, 2016b), this welfare 'reform' agenda has continued apace under the subsequent two Conservative governments. It has also included further intensification of benefit conditionality, initially a dramatic increase in the use of existing sanctioning powers (Watts et al., 2014), before a more severe formal regime was introduced from 2012, including an unprecedented maximum sanction of complete benefit withdrawal for three years.

Thus, concerns about welfare dependency reached fever pitch on both sides of the Atlantic in the 1980s and had clear policy impact from the 1990s onwards, despite a fierce academic and policy lobby arguing that this 'mythic' underclass did not exist (Bagguley and Mann, 1992; Dean and Taylor-Gooby, 1992; Lister, 1996; MacDonald, 1997). Paz-Fuchs (2008) notes that the moral(ising) agenda of promoting family values so explicit in the American debate on welfare conditionality was less prominent for New Labour, who instead foregrounded 'Third Way' ideas of 'social inclusion', influenced at least in part by ideas from Continental Europe (see below).

However, New Labour did share a political context with the US Clinton administration whereby centre-Left parties sought to establish their credential as 'tough on welfare'. The influence of the 'underclass' idea was more explicit in Conservative Prime Minister David Cameron's diagnosis of a 'broken society' characterised by high rates of teenage pregnancy, single parenthood and a dependency culture (see also Duncan-Smith, 2006; Centre for Social Justice, 2009, 2013). Under Theresa May's premiership there has been a rhetorical focus on those 'just managing', but there have only been only very limited signs of retreat from the welfare cutbacks instituted under her predecessor (the reversal of a policy on extending housing allowance restrictions operating in the private rented sector to social tenants being the sole significant example to date). There has been a substantial fall in levels of benefit sanctioning of Jobseeker's Allowance claimants since their historic peak in 2013 (National Audit Office, 2016), but the Universal Credit regime that is currently being rolled out will eventually replace most UK working-age benefits, and will see a further tightening of conditionality, including its controversial extension to the in-work benefits of those in low-paid employment (Dwyer and Wright, 2014). The passions aroused by these welfare dependency and conditionality debates also continue to be evident in the US: President Obama's decision to allow states to waive work-related requirements on welfare claimants prompted a furore (see Daguerre, 2013) and was subsequently reversed by President Trump (Office of Family Assistance, 2017), who has additionally initiated substantial cuts to the TANF grant which funds state welfare provision (Child Welfare League of America, 2017).

## *A need to activate? The European debate*

A different set of ideas have been important in galvanising support for conditionality across Continental Europe. The 'activation turn' describes a shift over the 1990s and 2000s, with longer-term roots going back to mid-twentieth-century Sweden, to reconcile the aims of social security with the reality of a dynamic and increasingly global economy and post-industrial labour market (Clasen and Clegg, 2006; Eichorst and Konle-Seidl, 2008; Keune and Serrano, 2013). According to Brodkin and Larsen (2013), activation, and the closely related ideas of workfare, welfare to work, work-first or 'insertion', combine compensatory, enabling and regulatory features.

The *compensatory* function refers broadly to 'passive' policies, or what might be considered 'classic' welfare state aims of smoothing income over the life course and/or redistributing it to those who are out of work in order to prevent hardship and poverty. The *enabling* and *regulatory* functions refer to two sides of the 'activation' coin: the former denotes policies that seek to 'pull' those who are out of work into work, including job search assistance, training schemes, in-work benefits and childcare support; the latter to policies that seek to 'push' people back into work by reducing the generosity of out-of-work benefits, placing time limits on benefit receipt, monitoring of job search efforts, and using sanctions to enforce these requirements.

An increased emphasis on welfare conditionality is, then, one crucial aspect of this activation turn, and the aspect which has perhaps the furthest-reaching consequences in altering the traditional 'decommodifying' role of the welfare state, i.e. the degree to which people can maintain an acceptable standard of living independently from the labour market (Clasen and Clegg, 2006). As noted in Chapter 1, however, Brodkin and Larsen (2013) distinguish between the European and a US 'path to workfare', with the latter characterised by a strong ideological agenda around welfare reliance as a moral failing, whereas European activation policies focused instead on balancing social protection with the desire to maintain full employment and ensure economic prosperity (Bonoli, 2010; Brodkin and Larsen, 2013). Denmark's 'flexicurity state' (Larsen, 2013) is seen to represent the apogee of this active labour market approach, which is now used widely across Europe, and supported by international agencies including the OECD and EU (Bonoli, 2010).

Thus, while something of a shift in the direction of the US-style hard-line workfare model has been discerned across Europe, important policy differences remain (see Chapter 3), not least with regard to sanctioning policies which range from imposing an initial 10% loss of benefit income in Germany, to 100% of benefit income for a 'first infringement' in the UK, and 'full-family' sanctions in the US. Likewise, while benefit sanctions last a standard three months in Germany (with repeat sanctioning possible) the maximum length of sanction in the UK is now three years, while in the US overall access to benefits is time-limited (Langenbucher, 2015; van den Berg et al., 2015).

## *Targeting young people*

Youth-targeting has been a key feature of activation policies across many developed economies, reflecting, in part, awareness of the particular vulnerability of young people to the impact of recession and the 'scarring' effects of experiencing unemployment during youth (Gregg and Tominey, 2005; Bell and Blanchflower, 2011; van den Berg et al., 2015; Pierson and Humpage, 2016). It may also possibly reflect their weaker electoral clout compared to older age groups, at least in those countries that lack compulsory voting (Smith, 2016). In Germany, for instance, under the Hartz reforms, unemployment assistance claimants under 25 are subject to tougher sanctions than older claimants (van den Berg et al., 2015). In 2014, the centre-Right Abbot government in Australia announced new measures to impose a six-month waiting period on benefit claimants under 30 years old. After six months in receipt of benefits, it was proposed that young people would face another six-month exclusion, with the cycle continuing until the claimant gained employment, entered full-time education or turned 30. Strong resistance led to a softened measure being introduced, imposing a one-off four-week wait on work-ready under-25-year-olds (with some exemptions), and requiring them to participate in a 'rapid activation strategy' involving additional work search activities (Thomas, 2016). The expressed aim of the measure was to 'set the clear expectation that young people must make every effort to maximise their chances of successfully obtaining work' (Australian Government, 2015, p.27).

Activation schemes specifically targeting young people have also been a feature of UK policy, with the mandatory New Deal for Young People introduced in 1998 to help move young people who had been out of work for six months into employment (Pierson and Humpage, 2016). The 2010 Coalition government replaced the various New Deal programmes with the Work Programme, covering all long-term unemployed people, and the 2015 Conservative government announced a Youth Obligation targeting all out-of-work 18- to 21-year-olds. The aims of this programme have clear echoes with both the enabling aspects of activation policies and the underclass narratives discussed above:

> We are determined to fulfil our commitments to end the welfare culture that is embedded in some of Britain's most vulnerable communities. By working across government to make sure that every young person is in work or training, by opening up 3 million more apprenticeships, expanding traineeships, and making sure that a life on benefits is simply not an option, we want to end rolling welfare dependency for good, so welfare dependency is no longer passed down the generations.
>
> *(Cabinet Office, 2015)*

Young people subject to the Youth Obligation (being implemented on a phased basis from April 2017) are subject to increased conditionality from 'day one'. Required to take part in a three-week Intensive Activity Programme (or 'boot camp') to enhance their work-readiness, those who remain out of work after six months must take up an apprenticeship, training or community work placement to continue receiving benefits (Cabinet Office, 2015; House of Commons Work and Pensions Committee, 2017).

Regardless of any such specific targeting of conditionality on young benefit claimants, there is international evidence that this group are much more likely to receive sanctions than older claimants (Pavetti et al., 2003; Peters and Joyce, 2006; Watts et al., 2014; Reeves and Loopstra, 2017). However, it is not clear whether this association reflects less willingness or concern amongst young people to comply with work-related conditions; greater vulnerability and higher support needs amongst the younger cohort of unemployed people; or discrimination of some kind (deliberate or unconscious) on the part of those administering these systems (Watts et al., 2014).

## *Expanding the reach to sick and disabled people*

A key feature of the activation turn has been the extension of its mechanisms, including conditionality, to a broader group of 'work-less' individuals, notably sick and disabled people deemed capable of work or work-related activity (Clasen and Clegg, 2007). This extension in the scope of conditionality has occurred across Anglosphere countries, Scandinavia and Western Europe, justified by national governments and the OECD on the basis that it helps reduce claimant rates, and benefits sick or disabled claimants themselves in terms of their income, health and broader 'social inclusion' (Geiger, 2017). Hultqvist and Nørup (2017) argue that in the Nordic context this reflects a 'narrowing' of the idea of social inclusion from one covering various domains to one concerned overridingly with labour market participation.

In his international review, Geiger (2017) identifies a range of differences in the ways countries design and implement conditionality targeting disabled people. Many follow a rehabilitation-before-access model, in which disabled claimants remain on 'mainstream' out-of-work benefits, but with conditionality requirements re-focused on engagement with rehabilitation-focused support and/or work-related activity. Some version of this approach applies in Australia, Norway, Sweden and Denmark. After some period on this augmented conditionality regime (18 months in Australia and a year in Norway) claimants can seek access to a less behaviourally conditional (or 'unconditional') disability benefit or 'pension'.

In the UK, by contrast, sick/disabled claimants immediately seek access to the sickness benefit (Employment and Support Allowance, ESA) via a 'functional capacity test'. Introduced in 2008 and targeting recipients of incapacity benefits with overt work-related conditionality for the first time in the UK context (Dwyer et al., 2016), ESA distinguishes between three broad groups: those deemed capable of work, who will remain subject to full conditionality on the main out-of-work benefit, Jobseeker's Allowance; those who will be subject to a lower-level of conditionality while receiving ESA (the Work-Related Activity Group); and those whose condition warrants complete exemption from conditionality (the ESA Support Group). This assessment and classification process has generated significant controversy since its introduction, particularly on grounds that people for whom employment is not a realistic prospect are being classified as 'fit for work' or work-related activity, putting them at higher risk of sanction, with potentially significant negative material and psychological impacts (Baumberg et al., 2015; Barr et al., 2016; and see Chapter 5).

Geiger (2017) argues that the implementation of conditionality for this group can be understood on two dimensions – the emphasis on rehabilitation and associated support, and the stringency of conditionality – resulting in a four-quadrant categorisation. In the first quadrant, '*demanding*' models combine high conditionality with intensive rehabilitation, with Denmark the exemplar here. Mandatory rehabilitation activities in Denmark can include a 'work trial' to assess future capacity to work, or a one- to five-year 'Resource Activation' rehabilitation programme. Alternatively, Danes with extremely limited capacity to work can enter the 'Flex-Job' scheme of subsidised employment, in which they may face requirements to work as little as one to two hours per week (Hultqvist and Nørup, 2017; Geiger, 2017). '*Passive*' models combine low conditionality with weak rehabilitation, and Geiger identifies Norway and Germany as in this category, given research regarding the weak implementation of what are on paper highly activating policies. The UK (and to a lesser extent Australia) exemplifies a '*compliance-based*' system, which combines high conditionality with weak rehabilitation, pushing – but not supporting – disabled claimants into work (Patrick, 2011; Dwyer et al., 2016). The final potential characterisation constitutes a '*low conditionality, high rehabilitation*' regime. Though none of the cases considered by Geiger fit this category, Sweden's 'autonomy focused' approach to conditionality for this group is a likely contender (see Hultqvist and Nørup, 2017).

Crucially, Geiger's review suggests that while requirements are commonly applied to this group, sanctions are only rarely employed in practice (this is the case in Germany, the Netherlands, Denmark, Norway and Sweden). Australia and the UK are exceptions in this regard, applying sanctions to substantial numbers of sick and disabled benefit claimants. In Australia, an estimated one quarter of all imposed sanctions fall on disabled claimants (around 150,000 sanctions were applied to this group in just the first quarter of 2016) (Geiger, 2017). In the UK, while sanctions rates of those on ESA run well below those experienced by JSA recipients, it is estimated that around 400,000 ESA claimants have been sanctioned since 2008, with a quarter of such sanctions lasting over three months. Those with 'mental and behavioural' conditions fare worst of all (although more recent measures have sought to address this, with some success) (Geiger, 2017; Webster, 2017). Combined with sanctioning of JSA claimants with a disability, it is estimated that around 90,000 disabled people a year experience a sanction in the UK, and that disabled JSA claimants are at considerably higher risk of being sanctioned than their non-disabled counterparts (Geiger, 2017).

## Low-income families with children

As discussed above, workless lone parents have long been a main target of employment-related conditionality in the US. Recent years have also seen work-related conditionality extended to lone parents with children above an incrementally reducing age threshold in the UK. Since 2012, single out-of-work parents with a youngest child aged five or above have faced work-related requirements similar to those facing childless claimants, though with some 'flexibilities' (to work part-time within school hours, for instance) (Johnsen, 2016). This youngest-child age threshold was subsequently reduced to the age of three in 2017 (Dewar and Ben-Galim, 2017), bringing the UK into line with the

position in France, Germany, Norway and Switzerland (Finn and Gloster, 2010; Haux, 2013). In some US states and Canadian provinces the age of the youngest child at which work-related conditions apply can be much lower again (under one), while in a number of countries the age at which conditionality applies is decided at the discretion of case managers (Finn and Gloster, 2010).

Parallel to these trends, since the late 1990s, a much broader range of conditional welfare programmes targeting low-income families with children has also emerged, across both the developed and developing world, with the behavioural responses sought not only, or even primarily, in the labour market sphere, but rather mainly in the realms of education, health and child protection.

The most prominent manifestation of this trend can be found in the conditional cash transfer (CCTs) schemes, now found fairly widely across the Global South, following the first national CCT programme *Oportunidades*, introduced in Mexico in 1997. There are now also examples of CCTs in Europe (European Commission, 2014) and North America (Fiszbein et al., 2009). Such programmes aim to improve health and education outcomes, and alleviate poverty, in the short term by providing cash transfer payments and seeking to stimulate demand for public services (Pellerano and Barca, 2014). But there is also an ambition to improve outcomes in the long run via these programmes, including inter-generationally, by making those transfers 'conditional on pre-specified investment in household human capital' (Kabeer et al., 2012, p.4).

Typically, requirements of CCTs include that parents enrol children in school and ensure their attendance, vaccinate children and/or participate in regular health checks and nutrition education sessions (Bastagli, 2009; Barrientos, 2011). Payments are usually made to mothers, though sometimes to fathers or children/young people directly, and range from very small additions to household income to significant contributions increasing household income by 20–30% (Fernald et al., 2008). Schools and health clinics typically verify that requirements have been met, although in Chile the *Solidario* programme involves social workers helping families develop an action plan, with benefit receipt attached to its implementation (Kabeer et al., 2012). Similarly, in Brazil, non-compliance with conditions can lead to a visit from a social worker to explore whether beneficiaries are facing barriers to participation in education/health programmes, with a view to helping them resolve any such barriers (Fiszbein et al., 2009). Sanctions generally comprise a temporary reduction in benefit, sometimes followed by termination of the benefit for repeated non-compliance (Fiszbein et al., 2009). Programmes vary from the small scale – targeting, for instance, poor rural areas – to national programmes covering high proportions of families (40% of households in Ecuador, and 11 million families in Brazil according to Kabeer et al., 2012).

There are parallels between CCTs and the employment-focused behavioural conditionality agenda considered above, specifically with regard to concerns about 'welfare dependency' and the implications for economic productivity. In a systematic review of evidence on CCTs, Kabeer et al. (2012) explain:

> It is argued that tying cash transfers to human capital investments in children will help to break the inter-generational transmission of poverty by increasing their productivity as adults. This in turn will help to counter the view held by many governments and donors that social transfers are unproductive and give rise to welfare dependence on the part of recipients.
>
> *(p. 4)*

But there are also important differences. Aside from the much broader reach of these programmes, into the education, health and child welfare spheres, rather than simply labour market behaviours, CCTs can be interpreted as operating more as an incentive-based than sanctions-backed form of conditionality (though admittedly this distinction is not accepted by all; see Chapter 2). It is the promise of gains in the absence of pre-existing welfare support structures, rather than the threat of deprivation in the context of a well-established welfare system, that seeks to shift behaviour. There is therefore a distinction to be drawn, we would argue, between the introduction or ramping up of behavioural conditions within extant benefits systems, and the introduction of CCTs as part of an attempt to establish social protection systems where none have previously existed or they are very rudimentary. CCTs are further distinct in that the 'human development' agenda is fundamental and constitutive of their aims and design.

Conditional welfare programmes that reach beyond labour market behaviours in targeting low-income families are not limited to the developing economies, but have been a key feature of recent social policy in Australia in particular, and also in some of the other advanced welfare states. In the US, for example, PRWORA introduced Individual Responsibility Plans – contracts between states and claimants – that could include requirements (enforced by benefit withdrawal) to ensure claimants' children's school attendance, immunisation and engagement with appropriate substance misuse treatment (Paz-Fuchs, 2008). A measure operating in France from 2010 enabled the suspension of family benefits in cases of persistent truancy, though it was found to violate the Revised European Social Charter under the European Committee of Social Rights Collective Complaints procedure (EUROCEF, 2012) and was repealed in 2013. Similar proposals were mooted in the UK under the previous Blair (Hayden and Blaya, 2005) and Cameron (HM Treasury, 2015) administrations. There has also been recent consideration (though ultimately not pursued) of an extension in the aims of benefit conditionality to mandate people who have drug or alcohol problems, or who are obese, to address these health and lifestyle issues, albeit with a view mainly to labour market integration (Department for Work and Pensions, 2015; Black, 2016).

While, alongside the US and UK, Australia introduced welfare conditionality targeting unemployed people in the late 1990s (the 'Work for the Dole' programme) (Crisp and Fletcher, 2008), according to Taylor et al. (2016) child welfare – rather than primarily labour market participation – has provided 'both the impetus and the political justification for the implementation of new conditionality' (p.8). Three key developments are particularly worthy of note here.

First, in the late 1990s, in response to concerns about low immunisation rates, childcare benefits and lump sum maternity payments for new parents in Australia became conditional on proof of age-appropriate immunisations. Such conditionality remains part of the administration of Family Tax Benefits, and recent government announcements have expressed an intention to tighten existing limited exemptions to these requirements (Taylor et al., 2016).

Second, in 2009, the School Enrolment and Attendance through Welfare Reform Measure (SEAM) enabled parents' receipt of a wide range of income support payments to be made conditional on their children attending school, taking inspiration from similar developments in the US (see above). The measures were targeted in the Northern Territories, forming part of a wider set of emergency responses to an inquiry into the welfare of Aboriginal children (Taylor et al., 2016). SEAM was explicitly justified as aiming 'to foster responsibility and provide a platform for people to move up and out of welfare dependence' (Macklin, 2009, cited in Taylor et al., 2016, p.13).

Third, and most controversial, are Australia's compulsory income management policies wherein a proportion (often 50% but up to 90%) of a claimant's income support is paid via a BasicsCard, which can only be used in approved stores and cannot be spent on alcohol, tobacco, pornography or gambling (Taylor et al., 2016; Bray et al., 2014). They are thus of a slightly different structure to 'classic' conditional programmes, in that access or continued receipt is not dependent on particular behaviour or actions. Rather, particular actions (the purchase of certain goods) is restricted by the mechanism of delivery. Income management was first introduced in 2007 to parts of the Northern Territories and has since been expanded across Australia. Claimants can be subject to income management if they: have been referred as vulnerable by a social worker, child protection authority, or (in Queensland) the Family Responsibilities Commission; have clinically diagnosed alcohol issues; are 15–24 years old and have been claiming benefits for three of the last six months; or are over 24 and have been claiming benefits for over 12 of the last 24 months. The introduction of income management, like SEAM, followed an inquiry into the welfare of Aboriginal children and was initially compulsory for claimants in specific Indigenous communities only, requiring the disapplication of anti-discrimination legislation. Subsequent reforms have widened the applicability of income management measures, though the vast majority of those affected continue to be Indigenous people.

The primary rationale given for these income management measures was to protect benefit recipients' children from abuse, maltreatment and generally poor outcomes associated with problem drinking and irresponsible parenting, by ensuring that 'income support payments are allocated in beneficial ways [and . . .] that the first call on welfare payment should be life essentials and the interests of children' (Australian Government, 2009, p.1). But it has been found that over half of those subject to income management do not have dependent children (Bray et al., 2014), suggesting that the programme in reality seeks to 'responsibilise' the spending of a wider group of people than just parents.

In their review of 'New Conditionality' in Australia, Taylor et al. (2016) comment that, while there has been broad support for conditionality targeting immunisation and school enrolment and attendance, income management has proved extremely controversial, seen by some as unjustifiably paternalistic, stigmatising and discriminatory against Indigenous Australians (Bielefeld, 2012). Compulsory income management targeting 16- to 18-year-old benefit recipients in New Zealand has been similarly controversial (Humpage, 2016), as have proposals in the UK (not pursued to date) to introduce a pre-paid 'yellow card' as a 'non-financial sanction' for those failing to meet conduct requirements associated with their benefits (Miscampbell, 2014, p.7).

## Social tenants

Housing, particularly social or public housing, can operate as a key site for conditional forms of welfare, wherein the prospect of losing one's home, or being barred from accessing one in the first place, may be viewed as a particularly powerful sanction encouraging or compelling desired behavioural patterns (Fitzpatrick and Watts, 2017; Flint et al., 2011). It is also a welfare domain within which conditionality can be argued to have increased in recent years, especially in the UK and Australia. Housing-related behavioural conditionality takes two main forms: first, *allocations policies* of landlords that include behavioural criteria in determining who can access social housing; second, *tenancy law* and policies which employ behavioural criteria in determining the length of time for which existing tenants can retain their social tenancy.

The UK retains a comparatively large social rented sector by international standards, accounting for about one in six of all dwellings (Wilcox et al., 2017). However, recent shifts towards more conditional approaches in the social housing sphere, in England specifically, mark a (partial) departure from two established characteristics of previous policy: first, from a needs-based allocation system, established in the 1970s, in explicit rejection of earlier desert-based approaches (Fitzpatrick and Stephens, 1999); and, second, from security of tenure, dating from 1980, which meant that tenants had indefinite right to occupy their homes unless they breach their tenancy agreement (Fitzpatrick and Stephens, 2007).

The erosion of the security of tenure of English social tenants first began with the introduction, in 1996, of 'probationary' tenancies by the then Conservative government, which meant that full security of tenure could be delayed for new social tenants (for up to 18 months), and then by the implementation of 'demoted' tenancies in 2003, by the then Labour government, which reduced security for existing tenants subject to behavioural concerns (Garvie, 2012). While ministers of both main political parties also periodically suggested linking access to, and retention of, social housing tenancies to voluntary activities or work-seeking behaviour (see, for example, Caroline Flint, 2008), they did not follow through on this agenda until the Conservative-led Coalition government came to power in 2010.

The Coalition government's Localism Act 2011 left intact legal duties to give 'reasonable' priority in allocations to certain groups, including homeless households, but gave English councils new powers to restrict access to their housing waiting lists and encouraged them to give preference to various 'deserving' groups, such as those in work or making some other 'community contribution', and ex-services personnel (DCLG, 2012). More than half of English councils have taken up these 'flexibilities', leading to substantial reductions in the numbers of people on housing waiting lists (Barnes, 2016). Greater emphasis appears to have been placed on using these expanded powers to impose local residency requirements, rather than to reward job seeking or other 'pro-social' behaviour. This reflects in part strong government encouragement for local authorities to introduce two-year residency tests, but also the reluctance of local authorities of all political hues to introduce allocations procedures rewarding 'community contribution'. This reluctance stems from both practical concerns (about administration, and the definition and assessment of community contribution) and those of fairness, with many local authorities unwilling to prioritise desert over need and concerned about conflicts with equalities and human rights legislation (Conservative Home, 2012; Wilson and Barton, 2017).

The Localism Act also enabled social landlords in England to offer fixed-term (renewable) tenancies (usually for a minimum of five years) to new social tenants, with the government advising that income, employment status, under-occupancy and behaviour could all be taken into account in tenancy (non)renewal (Garvie, 2012). However, reflecting little enthusiasm on the part of many social landlords to restricting their tenants' security of tenure, only 15% of new social tenancies were let on a fixed-term basis by 2014/2015 (DCLG, 2016). The 2015 Conservative government was unhappy with this state of affairs and passed further legislation, in 2016, which – if and when brought into force – will make fixed-term tenancies mandatory for the vast majority of new local authority tenants (Fitzpatrick and Watts, 2017).

This shift towards expanded conditionality in social housing over the past two decades has been driven in part by a desire, especially prominent under Labour governments, to more effectively address 'anti-social behaviour' in social housing estates (Flint and Nixon, 2006). Family intervention projects designed to work with families with complex needs and behavioural issues have incorporated probationary tenancies – alongside intensive family support – which delay security of tenure for a specified period pending 'good behaviour' (Morgan, 2010; Flint, 2011). It has also been designed to address concerns, articulated particularly but not exclusively by Conservative politicians, that social housing fosters 'welfare dependency' and undercuts personal responsibility, particularly with respect to job seeking (Dwelly and Cowans, 2006; Greenhalgh and Moss, 2009; DCLG, 2012). However, at a time of acute pressure on a dwindling social housing stock, particularly in London and the south of England, the most influential rationale for increased conditionality seems to have been an 'equity' one (Fitzpatrick and Pawson, 2014), linked to an underlying conception of social housing as a 'welfare service' (Paris et al., 1985) whose occupants should be required to leave if their circumstances improve in order to free up this scarce resource for others in greater need (DCLG, 2010). This characterisation of the sector is fiercely resisted by many social landlords and others, and, in practice tackling under-occupation in pressurised market areas seems to be a main priority for social landlords voluntarily using fixed-term tenancies (Fitzpatrick and Watts, 2017). However, a small proportion of 'interventionist' housing associations appear to be using fixed-term tenancies to encourage, or even compel, their tenants to make a 'community contribution', for example through voluntary work, and/or make concerted efforts to find employment, or to address health and lifestyle issues (Fitzpatrick and Watts, 2017).

A combination of welfare dependency and equity rationales also appears to have informed the introduction of fixed-term social tenancies in Australia, starting in New South Wales in 2006, and now implemented in a number of other Australian states and territories (see, for example, State Government of Victoria, 2012). These developments provided the inspiration for the introduction of a similar model in England discussed above. Australia's very small public and community housing sector (less than 5% of stock) has, since the 1990s, been tightly targeted not only on low-income groups, but also those with additional special and/or complex social support needs (Fitzpatrick and Pawson, 2014). In practice, tenancy reviews at the end of fixed-term periods in Australia appear to focus on changes in tenant income, rather than the potentially much broader gamut of behavioural concerns discussed in the English context. In any case, almost all Australian fixed-term social tenancies seem to be renewed (Fitzpatrick and Pawson, 2014). This calls into question the purpose of the policy framework that seems destined to generate great insecurity and diminished work incentives for tenants, and a not inconsiderable administrative burden for landlords, with little by way of positive policy gain to show for it (Fitzpatrick and Pawson, 2014). Likewise, it has been argued in the English case that the likely very marginal welfare gains from fixed-term tenancies, in terms of increased turnover and a rise in available lettings, are heavily outweighed by detrimental impacts on both community stability and on the 'ontological' security of (mainly poor) social tenants (Fitzpatrick and Watts, 2017).

In the US and Canada, where the public housing sector is of a comparable scale to that in Australia, eligibility criteria is likewise drawn narrowly to focus on the lowest income groups, and those with additional support needs, with prioritisation amongst those who meet these strict criteria determined largely by date order waiting lists rather than by behavioural criteria (Fitzpatrick and Stephens, 2007). Tenancy arrangements vary between the various states in the US, and the provinces in Canada, but are generally on some kind of (renewable) fixed-term basis. As with Australia above, the US and Canadian public housing sectors have been characterised by Stephens (2008) as performing an 'ambulance service'-style temporary welfare function, reserved only for the very poorest on a highly conditional basis. However, Fitzpatrick and Pawson (2011) found that the income-related rents used by public landlords in North America were generally considered sufficient incentive for tenants whose circumstances improve to leave of their own accord without the need to formally end their lease on that basis. This same argument could equally be applied to Australia, where rents are also scaled to income (Fitzpatrick and Pawson, 2014), but UK government plans to force a similar 'pay to stay' policy on English local authorities were recently dropped (Apps, 2016).

It is not only in the English-speaking world that social housing has been a key site for conditional forms of welfare. In many European countries, including those with more highly redistributive 'social democratic' or 'corporatist' welfare regimes (Fitzpatrick and Stephens, 2014), and in some cases also large social rented sectors, considerations of behaviour and desert are a firmly entrenched feature of policy and practice. In their international review of social housing policy, including both Anglosphere and Continental European countries, Fitzpatrick and Stephens (2007) note that

> various groups of households are often excluded from mainstream social housing [across the developed economies]. These include people with rent arrears, or who seem likely to have difficulty in paying the rent, people with addiction or other behavioural problems, people with criminal records, and (in some countries) people with mental health problems. In many countries social landlords are also reluctant to house very-low-income households, or other vulnerable groups who are regarded as being poor risks. These people are often housed in a sub-sector

> of the social rented sector, which is generally cheaper and of lower quality than the mainstream sector, and lacks security of tenure.
>
> *(p.16)*

In Sweden, for example, municipal housing companies, who own almost one in five of all dwellings, are reluctant to allocate homes to those with low incomes or with additional support needs, in an approach which can be interpreted as almost the polar opposite of that in public housing in North America and Australia (Stephens et al., 2010; Scanlon et al., 2015). These disadvantaged groups are often instead accommodated in a 'secondary' housing market of sublet flats leased by Swedish local authorities, in which they lack security of tenure and face additional rules and requirements, for instance, concerning engagement with social service support plans and behavioural expectations (Sahlin, 2005; Olsson and Nordfelt, 2008). These highly conditional arrangements mirror a general tendency in Swedish public policy, as noted by Fitzpatrick and Stephens (2014), to ally a renowned commitment to egalitarianism with an exceptionally strong regard for social cohesion, behavioural conformity and personal responsibility, such that marginalised groups whose conduct transgresses societal norms (Jenks, 2003) can find the barriers to assistance very high.

Similarly, France and Austria's 'very social' housing sectors cater for those on very low incomes, out of work and otherwise marginalised, and are characterised by less security of tenure than mainstream social housing, lower construction standards, social worker control over access, and concentration in disadvantaged areas (Levy-Vroelant and Reinprecht, 2014). Very social housing in France was explicitly designed as a behavioural tool to facilitate the reintegration or 'reinsertion' of its residents into society, achieved in part through conditional contracts linking residence to work search obligations. In Belgium, and to a lesser extent in Germany, there has been a significant growth since the 1980s in 'social rental agencies' which procure properties from the private sector to let to homeless people and other marginalised groups, such as those with mental health problems and ex-offenders, in part because households on the lowest incomes or with support needs or behavioural challenges are often excluded from the (very small) social rented sectors in these countries (De Decker, 2009; Stephens et al., 2010).

As can be seen from the above discussion, while some of the conditionality mechanisms deployed in the housing sphere pertain specifically to the fulfilment of tenancy agreements – namely to pay one's rent and desist from 'anti-social' forms of behaviour (Flint, 2011, 2015) – in some countries policy has either flirted with or implemented social housing-based sanctions that reinforce the labour market-based sanctions found in the social security system.

## Homeless people

Homeless people, particularly those involved in harmful and/or anti-social 'street culture' activities such as rough sleeping, substance misuse, street drinking and begging, are a key group targeted by conditional welfare interventions and other social control measures in many countries. While some faith-based and other homelessness organisations (Johnsen, 2014), as well as some academic commentators (Bowpitt et al., 2014), advocate approaches offering unconditional, 'non-judgemental sanctuary', there has been a recent shift across North America, Europe and Australia towards more 'interventionist' policies that explicitly seek behaviour change on the part of street homeless people. The relevant interventions span 'hard' *enforcement* action that seeks to compel those involved in rough sleeping and associated activities to change their lifestyles, to *coercive* measures that make access to housing and other forms of welfare conditional on desistance from certain forms of conduct, to 'softer' modes of *persuasion* seeking to encourage those targeted to engage with support (Johnsen et al., forthcoming).

### *Enforcement*

Enforcement-based measures, involving the use of national legislation or local ordinances to prohibit rough sleeping and related activities, are highly controversial across the developed world (USICH, 2012; Fernandez Evangelista and Jones, 2013; Johnsen et al., 2016; Watts et al., 2017). Measures 'criminalising' homelessness and associated behaviours are argued by NGOs to be increasing in European and American cities (Fernandez Evangelista and Jones, 2013; National Law Centre on Homelessness and Poverty, 2014), albeit that the criminalisation of 'vagrancy' and begging has a very long history (O'Sullivan, 2012), and the brutality of the treatment meted out to both homeless adults and street children in some developing world contexts has been well documented (Bhukuth and Ballet, 2015; Padgett and Priyam, 2017).

According to a National Law Centre on Homelessness and Poverty report (2014), 18% of the nearly 200 US cities surveyed had a city-wide ban on sleeping in public, with over a quarter prohibiting sleeping in specific public places, and over three quarters prohibiting begging in specific areas. FEANTSA (the European Federation of National Organisations Working with the Homeless) also highlight moves in this direction – albeit varied and uneven – in some European countries (Fernandez Evangelista and Jones, 2013). This agenda has been taken furthest in Hungary, where 2010 legislation enabled local authorities to prohibit homeless people habitually residing in public spaces, a power that was taken up by Budapest in early 2011 and justified by the mayor on the grounds that 'the purpose of the nation's capital, including the railway stations, the underpasses, and public spaces is not to allow people who have nothing to lose to continuously molest everyone else and to make Budapest unusable' (Misetics, 2013, p.104). It was later specified that violations of these ordinances twice in six months was punishable by a fine of around 500 Euros or imprisonment for up to 60 days. In 2011, rough sleeping was made illegal across the whole of Hungary, with a successful Constitutional Court challenge against these measures parried by an amendment to the constitution overturning the court's capacity to review such legislation. Despite these dramatic legal developments, the Hungarian measures do not seem to have been aggressively enforced (Misetics, 2013).

In England, begging is an arrestable offence under the Vagrancy Act of 1824, as is sleeping rough when an individual has been directed to and failed to take up a free place of shelter. The maximum penalty is a fine, and according to Johnsen and Fitzpatrick (2007), these powers were not extensively used for rough sleeping, though they were used to tackle begging in 'hot-spot' areas. Introduced in 1998, Anti-Social Behaviour Orders, or ASBOs (and successor orders introduced in 2014 legislation), seek to protect the public from behaviour causing 'harassment, alarm or distress', and can be used to place behavioural and/or geographical conditions on targeted individuals. Breaching these orders carries a maximum penalty of five years' imprisonment. Though they have a much wider remit than homelessness-related issues, ASBOs have been used to target rough sleeping and street drinking in some areas, as have the more recently introduced Public Spaces Protection Orders which enable local authorities to prohibit activities that have 'a persistent and unreasonable detrimental effect on the quality of life of those in the locality' (Sanders and Albanese, 2017). Johnsen and Fitzpatrick (2007, 2010) found that, when combined with individually tailored support, ASBOs and other enforcement interventions could prompt vulnerable individuals to engage with services, such as substance misuse programmes, and have 'life saving' results in some instances. But behavioural responses to these sorts of interventions were unpredictable and could instead result in the 'diversion' of vulnerable people into more dangerous activities and places, leading the authors to conclude that they represented a 'high risk strategy' (Johnsen and Fitzpatrick, 2007, p.ix; see also Chapter 5).

Other interventions often highlighted under the rubric of the 'criminalisation of homelessness' include anti-food-sharing laws, which restrict the distribution of food to homeless people (e.g. soup kitchens) in certain areas. Almost one in 10 (9%) of the US cities surveyed by the National Law Centre on Homelessness and Poverty (2014) had such restrictions in place. There have also been attempts in the UK (specifically in London) to restrict soup runs from certain rough sleeping hot-spots, though these have to date been unsuccessful given expectations of widespread resistance to such a move (Spurr, 2014). 'Designing out', also known as 'hostile', 'defensive' or 'disciplinary' architecture, involves the manipulation of the built environment to prevent or discourage street activity by, for instance, designing street furniture in a way that prevents it being slept on. Controversy about these architectural interventions reached a peak in the UK in 2014 when a photograph of alleged 'homeless spikes' outside a London office block went viral on Twitter, igniting widespread public outrage (Petty, 2016).

These enforcement interventions have, more generally, sparked significant opposition and activism defending the 'rights' of those targeted to use public space – their 'right to the city' (Attoh, 2011) or even their 'right to be homeless' (Coleman, 2000). Some scholars have described a 'revanchist urbanism' (Smith, 1996) seeking to 'eradicate', 'exterminate' or 'annihilate' the street homeless population in order to 'sanitise' the city in service to the needs of wealthy gentrifiers and global capital (Amster, 2003; Webb, 2014). However, it has been suggested that the 'polemical' claims of aggressive revanchism are overstated, at least in Europe and the UK (Tosi, 2007; Doherty et al., 2008; DeVerteuil et al., 2009; Johnsen and Fitzpatrick, 2010). Some working in the field see the selective deployment of enforcement measures as essential (and indeed a moral imperative) to address the physical, mental health and substance misuse challenges faced by the most vulnerable street homeless people (Swain, 2003; see also Watts et al., 2017). A 'compassionate thread' has been detected in enforcement-based responses to street homelessness in British cities (Johnsen and Fitzpatrick, 2010, p.15) and, based on an 'ethnographic revisit' to Los Angeles' Skid Row (the focus of Brittner's ethnography in 1967), Stuart (2014) argues that police draw on enforcement measures 'as a resource to "shepherd" homeless individuals into rehabilitative social services' (p.2). It seems, then, that local actor discretion is key to how enforcement-based approaches are implemented and the extent to which they are shaped to be compassionate and empowering, or to serve discriminatory and oppressive ends (Stuart, 2014; Potts and Martin, 2013; Johnsen and Fitzpatrick, 2007).

## *Conditionality and coercion*

Alongside an emphasis on force, to a greater or lesser degree, a high degree of conditionality is built into responses to street homelessness across the Global North, particularly in the traditional 'continuum of care' or 'treatment first' model that until very recently dominated both provision and thinking in the field. This approach sees homeless people moving through a series of emergency, transitional and supportive housing environments before accessing 'normal' housing only once they have demonstrated their 'housing readiness', and have addressed additional support needs, such as mental health or substance misuse problems (Johnsen and Texeira, 2010; Padgett et al., 2016; Sahlin,

2005; Gordon, 2008; Hansen Lofstrand, 2010; Levy-Vroelant and Reinprecht, 2014; Jones and Pleace, 2010).

The logic of this 'linear' approach hangs on the idea that those with experience of street homelessness need space to develop independent living skills, and to address health and other support needs, before taking on their own tenancy, and that supportive housing environments with sanction-backed behavioural expectations can provide an appropriate environment for them to do so. However, this model has been subject to substantial critique and challenge in recent years, as both ineffective at ending homelessness and having unintended exclusionary and institutionalising effects (Busch-Geertsema, 2014). The apotheosis of this approach may be found in Sweden's 'staircase of transition' (Sahlin, 2005), which has been argued to involve a degree of surveillance and social control over homeless people that would be considered unacceptable in more 'liberal', albeit less egalitarian, climates such as that found in the UK (Fitzpatrick and Stephens, 2014).

The highly influential Housing First model, first developed in the US but increasingly used across Europe and elsewhere in the developed world (Busch-Geertsema, 2014), departs radically from traditional 'linear' staircase approaches by promoting the rapid and permanent rehousing of vulnerable homeless people, alongside flexible and individualised 'wrap-around' support, without their having to first undergo treatment for mental illness or substance misuse problems (Tsemberis, 2010). It is based on an ethic of 'tolerance' quite distinct from that underpinning more conditional responses to homelessness, but does not imply a rejection of 'behaviour change' objectives. On the contrary, Housing First advocates an assertive and proactive approach to support that explicitly seeks to encourage homeless and vulnerable people away from self-destructive activities, such as engagement in substance misuse, and onto a sustained exit from homelessness (Johnsen and Teixeira, 2010). But engagement with this support (above a minimal level of contact) is not compelled and non-engagement does not put the service user's housing at risk. A wealth of evaluative evidence now demonstrates much higher levels of tenancy sustainment and other positive outcomes from Housing First approaches than the traditional staircase model (Padgett et al., 2016; Woodhall-Melnick and Dunn, 2016).

### *Persuasion*

In the US, UK and Australia there have also been shifts in the nature of street outreach services away from a traditionally 'ameliorative' approach to a more 'assertive' stance which overtly aims to persuade street homeless people to move into accommodation (Phillips et al., 2011). Though these assertive outreach models sometimes involve some elements of force or coercion, such as the compulsory 'Single Service Offer' now made to some rough sleepers in London (Hough et al., 2011), often they rely simply on the persistence and influencing skills of outreach workers, who are trained not to accept rejections of help as the final outcome. Such assertive approaches have been argued to be most defensible and effective where they are combined with the 'incentive' of a 'meaningful offer' of support and accommodation (Parsell, 2011), and rather more problematic where persistence and persuasion encourages those targeted to access services they may have legitimate reasons to avoid (e.g. related to concerns about their personal safety in congregate hostel settings). They have also been seen by some as in tension with social work principles of self-determination (Parsell, 2011), or with the ethos of some faith-based organisations concerned to provide unconditional hospitality and care (Johnsen, 2014; Johnsen and Jones, 2015).

Homelessness is thus a policy sphere in which the full range of social control mechanisms based on force, coercion and persuasion are brought to bear, as well as – and sometimes in combination with – tolerant, 'open door' responses that reject behaviour change objectives entirely (Johnsen et al., forthcoming). This sets the scene for heated policy and ethical debates (Watts et al., 2017; Johnsen et al., forthcoming). The romanticisation of rough sleeping as an alternative 'lifestyle choice', or claims that people have a 'right to be homeless', is given short shrift by some working in the sector who describe 'not a mutually supportive community but a disparate and wretched group of people forced together by circumstance, in need of a better life' (Swain, 2015, p.20; see also Parsell, 2011). Other stakeholders, however, are committed to the view that unconditional approaches offer the best prospect of successful outcomes with the most vulnerable homeless people, or maintain a principled objection to more interventionist models as in conflict with their faith-based commitments or an intuitively appealing 'ethic of care' (Bowpitt et al., 2014; Johnsen, 2014; Midgely, 2016). We seek to offer some tools to navigate the ethical dilemmas that suffuse these debates in Chapter 6.

## Concluding comments

Examples of conditional welfare now abound, seeking to promote specific behaviours amongst a range of target groups, not only in the advanced Western welfare states, but also in less economically developed countries. These conditional welfare policies are pursued by governments of both Left and Right, and across a wide range of 'welfare regime' types. This chapter has offered a selection of case studies of welfare conditionality targeted on unemployed people, young people, sick and disabled people, low-income families, social tenants and homeless people, in order to explore the range of 'problematic' behaviours targeted for intervention, the diversity of underpinning rationales, and the variety of mechanisms used.

The most well-known and well-documented focus of conditional welfare approaches has been the attempt to drive down unemployment, using sanction-backed work-related requirements within the social security system and, to a much smaller extent, the social housing system. But conditional welfare approaches are now pursued to tackle a much wider set of 'negative' behaviours and outcomes, from the spending of benefit income on 'non-essential' items, to poor school attendance and immunisation rates amongst children, to vulnerable adults' engagement in anti-social behaviour or harmful street lifestyles associated with rough sleeping, begging and substance misuse.

Threading through most of these targeted behaviours is a clear theme of seeking to minimise reliance on collective forms of welfare and bolster personal responsibility, as well as reduce social harms of various kinds. The spread and intensification of welfare conditionality has been widely interpreted, certainly in Anglosphere countries, as a *moral* agenda to reform the poor character of a welfare-dependent 'underclass', accompanied by a *regressive* agenda to promote the interests of (variously) global capital, neoliberalism and wealthy elites at the expense of poor or marginalised populations.

However, this narrative is to some degree challenged by the pursuit of behavioural conditionality in 'high tax, high spend' welfare regimes, where it has evolved to safeguard robust welfare safety nets in an increasingly competitive and open global market. It also fits less well with the development of conditional approaches in less economically developed countries, in Latin America and elsewhere in the Global South, where they have been core to the establishment and widening of a welfare safety net for poorer households. Furthermore, the well-being of the individuals targeted (or those in their care) is clearly a central motivation of some conditional welfare approaches, for example in the fields of child protection, family health and homelessness, but their socially controlling nature can nonetheless remain highly controversial.

The next chapter turns its attention to the impacts – intended and unintended, positive and negative – of these highly diverse forms of welfare conditionality, providing a firmer basis for our consideration of the multi-layered ethical dilemmas associated with conditionality in Chapter 6.

# 5

# THE IMPACTS OF CONDITIONALITY

This chapter reviews the empirical evidence on the impacts and outcomes of welfare conditionality, not only its efficacy as a technique in achieving programme goals but also the wider implications of its deployment for both those targeted by conditional interventions and broader society. It begins by examining the behavioural assumptions underpinning conditional welfare programmes, and critiques of these assumptions, which are intrinsic to the plausibility of the 'theory of change' underpinning the anticipated effects of such approaches. We then bring forward the existing evaluative evidence on the effectiveness of various techniques and programmes of conditional welfare, including from our UK-based *Welfare Conditionality* research programme, funded by the ESRC (see www.welfareconditionality.ac.uk; see also Chapter 1). We use this and other evidence to reflect on the potential unintended consequences of conditionality, taking into account relevant 'spill-over' and 'scar' effects, before moving on to a consideration of the issue of costs. Finally, we highlight the range of alternatives to welfare conditionality that exist as possible means to achieve behavioural change goals.

## Behavioural assumptions

In its reliance on (the threat of) sanctions or (promise of) incentives to bring about desired forms of behavioural change, welfare conditionality appears to rest on a particular set of assumptions about human motivation and agency. Specifically, that the behaviour of prospective or current welfare recipients is influenced by that person's rational assessment of the costs and benefits of particular courses of action. This aligns with an 'incentives paradigm' which sees 'a direct stimulus-response relationship between policy change and individual behaviour' (King, 2006, p.115).

Such perspectives reflect a view of human agency as reflexive, rational and intentional (Greener, 2002), and are associated with 'rational choice models', according to which 'the basic unit of society is the self-seeking individual motivated by their need and desire to maximise their own advantage' (Hudson and Lowe, 2009, p.225). Within welfare scholarship, this world view is reflected, for example, in Charles Murray's classic and controversial account (1984) of the development of an 'underclass' of single mothers who 'rationally' choose to become dependent on welfare payments, as a direct result of the perverse incentive structures provided by 'permissive' welfare institutions, as discussed in the last chapter.

Note that these rational choice models do not assume that people's *preferences* are 'rational' by some 'reasonable' external standard (Darnton, 2008). It is entirely consistent with such models that people may have tastes and preferences for things that harm them (e.g. smoking or eating unhealthy foods). They only require that people's preferences are consistent with each other and stable, and that, on the basis of those preferences, people act to maximise their 'utility', i.e. levels of 'happiness' or personal benefit (see also Chapter 6). Crucially, such models have also tended to assume that people have access to information relevant to the decision in question, and are able to understand and process that information effectively (Darnton, 2008).

While economists generally acknowledge that these assumptions are not literally true, their parsimony, applicability to a vast range of social and economic assumption, and claimed predictive power, have cemented their status as the fundamental building blocks of much public policy-making across the globe (Darnton, 2008; Hudson and Lowe, 2009; Hay, 2004; Australian Public Service Commission, 2007).

The implications of these models of behaviour for governments and policy-makers are clear: the welfare state can be thought of as a system of incentives and sanctions that will be assessed by potential and current recipients of those benefits and services in their rational calculations regarding how to behave. Thought of in this way, turning the dials on these incentives and sanctions using conditional forms of welfare offers policy-makers a lever to steer people's behaviour.

## *The challenge from behavioural economics*

The rational choice model of understanding human behaviour has been subject to extensive revision and critique, both within and beyond the economics discipline. Behavioural economics, a sub-discipline which seeks to ground economics in more realistic and plausible psychological insights about human beliefs and behaviour, has highlighted the 'bounded' nature of human rationality and the cognitive biases that characterise 'real life' decision-making processes (Simon, 1957; Tversky and Kahneman, 1974; Dawnay and Shah, 2005; King, 2006; Darnton, 2008; Australian Public Service Commission, 2007; Gibb, 2012).

Behavioural economists have emphasised, for example, that people make decisions in conditions of uncertainty, often under pressure, relying on heuristics or 'rules of thumb' rather than rational calculations (Tversky and Kahneman, 1974; Darnton, 2008). People tend to 'discount' the future, that is, attach higher value to short-term rather than long-term rewards. Those living 'impoverished and chaotic lives' have been shown to discount future utility particularly heavily, meaning that they are less likely to make longer-term investments in the financial, health, education or welfare realms (Halpern et al., 2004).

As Darnton (2008) points out, it is not necessarily the case that these heavier discounting rates are counter to self-interest: 'life expectancy is uncertain, investments are uncertain, health is uncertain' (p.8). Particularly given steep social gradients in health indicators, life expectancy and morbidity (Marmot, 2005; Aldridge et al., 2017), future discounting appears to be more rational for poorer than richer groups. It has also been argued that the experience of deprivation or 'scarcity' in itself creates a mind-set that makes it harder to process information and make good longer-term decisions (Mullainathan and Shafir, 2014), in part because decision-making styles develop specifically to cope with current stressful circumstances (Sheehy-Skeffington and Rea, 2017).

As discussed in Chapter 3, 'loss aversion' is a well-recognised psychological phenomenon, with people experiencing more 'pain' from the loss of a desired good than 'pleasure' at attaining an equivalent good (Dolan et al., 2012). Inertia is another important factor: faced with a difficult decision, people may not make a choice at all, or make the easiest choice (Darnton, 2008). This means that presenting or framing choices in specific ways – in a particular order, with a default option, or presenting the same options in terms of gains rather than losses – can make a significant difference to people's decision making (Cabinet Office/Institute for Government, 2010). It is the grain of these aspects of human decision making that 'nudge' models of behaviour change seek to work with (see Thaler and Sunstein, 2008, and discussion below).

These insights from behavioural economics must, however, be viewed as *augmenting* rather than negating rational choice models of human decision making and behaviour. As Jones et al. (2013) note, Kahneman and Tversky (two of the founding fathers of behavioural economics)

> [continue] to discern an essentially rational basis to human decisions ... heuristics and biases are not so much emotional aberrations as relatively predictable errors in attempts to make rational judgments under sub-optimal conditions.
>
> *(p.10)*

The goal of policy, for behavioural economists, then becomes to manage and correct these predictable irrationalities. The conception of human behaviour and decision making in terms of the metaphorical 'Homo Economicus' thus remains, 'if not as a reflection of actual human behaviour, then still as the paradigmatic goal' (Jones et al., 2013, p.10).

Behavioural economics does not therefore completely undercut the 'classic' rationale for welfare conditionality as a tool for behaviour change. On the contrary, an appreciation of people's bounded rationality and vulnerability to cognitive bias could, in fact, be thought to justify sanctions being used as a bargaining or coercive tool to *correct for* documented cognitive biases in human decision making. For instance, by imposing an immediate and substantial financial sanction on someone for failing to actively seek work, welfare systems may be argued to promote the welfare of disadvantaged groups who systematically 'under-value' the medium- to long-term benefits of obtaining work – a higher income over the life course – relative to the short-run benefits of not working (see, for example, the arguments of Lawrence Mead, 1986, discussed in Chapter 4). Moreover, the fact that people in general tend to be more concerned to avoid losses than they do to seek equivalent gains may indicate that sanctions (for job search failures) rather than incentives (rewarding job search efforts) are the more effective way to intervene in such cases (Jensen et al., 2003; Dolan et al., 2012; cf. Jochelson, 2007). Against this, drawing on the 'scarcity mind-set' research discussed above, Curchin (2017; see also Oliver, 2013) has argued that behavioural science insights 'can be used to mount a case for a more generous, less punitive approach to income support' (p.243). She explains:

> Behaviour research reveals that counter-productive behaviour is to be expected when people are placed in circumstances hostile to their well-being. Rather than locate the deficit within individuals, it locates it within the context of scarcity in which some individuals are forced to live. This points not to a need to remedy the character of individuals – rather it suggests the importance of remedying social conditions.
>
> *(p.233)*

## More fundamental challenges

More thoroughgoing critiques of the allegedly 'seductively simple' (Wright, 2012) rational actor model can, however, be found outside of economics. Models of human agency have been developed by scholars in the sociology and social policy disciplines in particular that foreground the non-rational underpinnings of human behaviour and the role of impulse, passion and emotion.

In his postmodern account, Zygmunt Bauman (1993), for example, emphasises the importance of internal and external contradictions and ambivalence, and the role of irrational impulses and sympathies in underpinning human action, commenting that 'people do things which would hardly pass the test of an accountable, let alone "reasonable", purpose' (p.33). Coming from a very different perspective, Steven Lukes suggests an understanding of both people's subjective preferences and their 'real interests' as multiple and contradictory (Lukes, 2005), while Paul Hoggett (2001), drawing on psychoanalytic theory, argues for a non-unitary conception of 'the self' as potentially 'split' or fragmented:

> we are several selves, each characterised by a different voice and a different mood, some of which we identify with and feel close to, some of which seem unfamiliar and alien. Which self or part of us dominates at any moment in time and initiates action or makes choices depends upon the social relations we engage in and the roles we take up. It is because the self that acts or chooses may be unfamiliar to us that it is possible to say that we do not always know why we do what we do.
>
> *(p.41)*

Such complex and fragmented accounts of human agency and motivation suggest that decision making is likely to depart – potentially quite radically – from that predicted by traditional rational actor models, and even from the imperfect rationality captured in the accounts of behavioural economists. They therefore cast doubt on the predictability and reliability of achieving desired behavioural outcomes through incentives and sanctions. From this perspective, such behaviour-change mechanisms will 'work' only sometimes and often be ineffective. At worst, they risk leading to a range of unintended and potentially highly undesirable behavioural and other outcomes.

These perspectives have commonly been used in critiques of welfare conditionality. Wright (2012), for instance, argues that human agency is best understood as:

> contextual, emergent, contingent, relational and dynamic, rather than strictly individual, unitary, rational or purposive ... [and that this] presents a fundamental challenge to several aspects of the existing model of agency enshrined in UK welfare-to-work policies [and] the carrot and stick approach of behavioural instrumentalism.
>
> *(p.324)*

## *Finding a middle ground*

These starkly opposing perspectives on human agency each have obvious limitations. Rational actor theories, at first glance, appear to rest on the 'absurd assumption of perfect rationality' (Somerville and Bengtsson, 2002, p.124), as well as unrealistic notions of human actors having unlimited access to information and boundless capacities to efficiently process this information. However, such a critique is somewhat to miss the point. As noted above, those who employ classic economic rationality assumptions seldom claim that they are literally true: they are not concerned with the 'descriptive realism' (Darnton, 2008, p.6) of these assumptions but rather with their analytical power, that is, their capacity to explain or predict behavioural outcomes. These assumptions are acknowledged to represent an oversimplified view of the world and advocates of the standard rational actor model point out that, despite their obvious limitations, they have considerable utility in providing 'powerful insights for human behaviour' (Darnton, 2008, p.6; see also Harford, 2008). Rationality assumptions have underpinned the success of numerous public policy interventions encouraging pro-social behaviours, with examples ranging from traffic congestion charges (Darnton, 2008), to levies on plastic bags (Australian Public Service Commission, 2007), to the raising of taxes on tobacco, alcohol and sugar (Mirrlees, 2010). Moreover, the 'extreme' critiques of economic understandings of human agency appear to ignore the major strides taken in behavioural economics and allied disciplines, which go a considerable way to explaining seemingly non-rational or irrational behaviour (Darnton, 2008; Cabinet Office/Institute for Government, 2010; Dolan et al., 2012).

Thus, while perspectives that highlight the role of emotion, impulse, irrationality and multiplicity of motivation are a necessary counterpoint to hubristic over-reliance on a rigidly 'economistic' worldview, in some instances they seem to seriously overstate the case against rational actor models and their behavioural descendants.

Perspectives that emphasise the non-rational or irrational aspects of human decision making also have a further limitation. Namely, that they fail to offer a useful framework for *predicting* behaviour – a crucial ingredient in anticipating the impact of social policies. Though they may go some way to explaining why behavioural conditionality may not 'work' as we expect it to, they are perhaps less helpful in offering models of decision making that can be used to inform policy design to achieve specific ends.

Taken to its logical conclusion, a particularly unproductive interpretation of this stance would be that people's behaviour is wholly irrational, unpredictable and impervious to external stimuli, and thus it is futile for policy-makers, short of the deployment of actual force, to attempt to shape the decisions that atomistic individuals make, even where they are harmful to themselves or others. As well as lacking utility as a framework to inform policy-making, such a perspective risks representing the users of welfare policy as entirely lacking in the capacity for self-determination (see Deacon and Mann, 1999) – buffeted as they are by the wild winds of impulse, emotion and irrationality.

A route out of this fix is offered by an applied 'theory of the middle range', with its roots in social theory (Elster, 1983) and (more recently) housing studies (Somerville and Bengtsson, 2002), which suggests that behaviours, decisions and choices that may *appear* irrational or impulsive may nevertheless be 'rational' when viewed in context of the 'actor in focus' (a perspective that is not as far removed from that of traditional economic models than some of its advocates may be willing to concede). From this viewpoint

> individual actors are assumed to have some logical consistency in the pursuit of their goals, whereas the nature of those goals (the preferences of the actors, including the social norms they adhere to) is not assumed a priori by the researcher but is open to

> empirical investigation, where the social and institutional context is of crucial importance.
>
> *(Somerville and Bengtsson, 2002, p.124)*

For example, in his consideration of the American 'ghetto' and critique of social inquiry into urban poverty, Wacquant emphasises the importance of understanding 'that forms of social action and organisation that may appear deviant, "aberrant", or downright inexplicable from afar (and above) obey a local social rationality that is well suited to the real-life constraints and facilitations of the contemporary Black Belt' (1997, p.348). Similarly, Nicholls (2009) argues that 'transgressive acts' (Jenks, 2003) by street homeless people, including resistance to engagement with support, alcohol misuse and street sex work have their own rationality and can be understood as 'the "best" option, however damaging, for these people, given the context they operated within' (Nicholls, 2009, p.77, see also Nicholls, 2010).

This idea of 'thin rationality' seems particularly useful in offering a framework within which to interpret welfare recipients' responses to behavioural conditionality where they may at first sight appear non-rational. In such cases, a concerted attempt to perceive the pay-offs and costs at issue from 'inside' the world view from which they are actually experienced will likely pay dividends. Seeing agency in this way – as *contextually rational* – also leaves ethical space for policy and service providers to attempt to enhance welfare service users' personal autonomy by fostering their 'capacity to set [their] own ends or purposes according to some rational standard' (Grant, 2006, p.34), as further discussed in Chapter 6.

There is thus ample room within this 'middle range' theory of agency for accounts that 'translate' apparently irrational behaviour into explicable reactions to the strong influence of people's environment and context. There is also space to incorporate the findings of increasingly influential work on the impact of 'adverse childhood experiences' (including abuse, neglect and other forms of household dysfunction) on health and wellbeing in later life (Bellis et al., 2014). For those with the most adverse childhood experiences, these impacts can lead to impulsive, non-rational behaviour when individuals are exposed to 'stressors' or 'triggers' in adulthood. These insights are increasingly recognised to be fundamental to effective service design in working with highly vulnerable populations – for example, those experiencing entrenched homelessness (Theodorou and Johnsen, 2017) – and we would argue have important applications in considering the efficacy of conditional forms of welfare (do such approaches help or hinder engaging with and addressing the needs of these groups?).

Such perspectives alert us to the possibility that approaches to behavioural change employing rewards and sanctions will not always be effective. First, the well-established information and capacity constraints, heuristics and cognitive biases documented by the behavioural sciences may interrupt classic 'pay-off' structure reasoning, though conditional interventions could be designed to counter these effects, or work with the grain of them. Second, by understanding rationality as potentially 'thin' or 'socially embedded', particularly as exercised by marginalised or disadvantaged groups, it is acknowledged that decisions and behaviour may be unpredictable or inexplicably from 'above' (to paraphrase Wacquant) and un-generalizable to whole populations. Third, for some population groups, past adverse experiences and present-day 'triggers' may *on occasion* combine to elicit genuinely irrational or non-rational responses.

This more nuanced account of agency does not, however, require us to completely dispense with the idea that people's conduct is shaped to a large degree by some form of 'rationality' and indeed, very often by 'economistic' reasoning. But this account does imply caution in *assuming* the effectiveness of welfare conditionality in bringing about desired forms of behavioural change. So it is to this question of the effectiveness in practice of welfare conditionality that we now turn our attention.

## Effectiveness

The major empirical question in this field is whether welfare conditionality 'works', i.e. does it bring about desired forms of behavioural change? Obvious follow-up questions include whether any relevant behavioural change is achieved in a cost-effective manner, with the relevant 'costs' defined to encompass unintended as well as intended consequences, as compared with the available alternatives? These supplementary questions are dealt with later in the chapter. Here we focus our attention on the available evidence on whether behavioural conditionality 'works' on its own terms.

We hope to demonstrate in this section that there can be no single answer to the question 'does conditionality work?', either in theory (as so much depends on one's objectives, context and the specific mechanisms used) or in practice (given the highly variable findings of available empirical evidence). However, it is possible to derive some key overarching lessons and messages from the wealth of data and studies now available.

In seeking to assess the efficacy of different forms of welfare conditionality, it is important to first acknowledge the sheer diversity of welfare realms within which this collection of techniques are now exercised, and also the unevenness in the quality and completeness of the evaluative evidence available on the effectiveness of these interventions.

To take a pertinent example from one end of this evidence spectrum, systematic evaluation of the efficacy of CCTs has been core to their development and implementation, often involving large-scale randomised control trials (RCTs) (Fiszbein et al., 2009). For instance, the *Oportunidades* programme in Mexico was introduced using an RCT methodology to test its effectiveness, and an expansive volume of literature has subsequently emerged assessing the impact of CCTs elsewhere (Kabeer et al., 2012; Fiszbein et al., 2009). This body of evidence indicates that well-designed CCTs that attend to context (Bastagli, 2009) can be effective in achieving programme outcomes (e.g. Fiszbein et al., 2009; Kabeer et al., 2012). For example, considerable evidence demonstrates the effectiveness of CCTs in increasing school enrolment and attendance, and also reductions in child labour (though evidence on impacts of these programmes on educational attainment is less definitive) (Pellerano and Barca, 2014).

Lively and at times controversial debate endures, nonetheless, about the added value of explicit conditionality over unconditional cash transfers (UCTs) (Pellerano and Barca, 2014; Kidd, 2016). UCTs have also been shown to have positive effects on the outcomes sought by CCTs, including, for instance, children's participation in education. A systematic review of 35 studies showed that CCTs and UCTs *both* had significant impacts on school enrolment levels, though the scale of impacts was generally greater for CCTs, especially when compliance was monitored and non-compliance penalised (Baird et al., 2014). However, in a more recent review of experiments comparing UCTs and CCTs in several African countries, Kidd (2016) concludes that there is as yet no definitive evidence on the added value of CCTs over UCTs.

The unevenness of these conclusions in part reflects the fact that much depends on the context for, and design of, such programmes (see also Bastagli, 2009). Fiszbein et al. (2009), for instance, explain that the appropriate choice of UCT or CCT will depend on *why* families are not sending their children to school. If families are choosing not to send children to school because they know the quality of education provided is poor, and there is more to be gained for both the family and the child by staying at home and (in their example) 'learning how to tend the fields or how to weave a basket with their parents' (p.46), CCTs may impose heavy and inefficient burdens on families, who will either comply, but with little benefit accruing to them, their child or wider society, or *not* comply and face sanctions (potentially causing greater vulnerability; see Rossel et al., 2017). If, on the other hand, families are underestimating the benefits of sending their children to school, the incentives offered by CCTs may result in behavioural shifts highly beneficial to the household and wider society.

There is also now a great deal of evidence and debate regarding the efficacy of sanctions-backed forms of behavioural conditionality in developed welfare state benefit systems, albeit that this evidence is often patchy and inconclusive, or even contradictory, and seldom based on RCTs (see Griggs and Evans, 2010; MacVicar, 2014; Ray et al., 2014; Geiger, 2017 for reviews). Nonetheless, a number of key lessons do emerge from studies from across the US, UK, Europe and Australia that can be summarised here.

First, there is no doubt that strict sanctioning regimes can dramatically reduce the numbers claiming welfare benefits. The clearest example of this is in the US, where the 1996 introduction of the highly conditional TANF programme precipitated a massive decline in welfare programme caseloads, albeit in combination with the impacts of a growing economy and employment opportunities

(Ray et al., 2014). After reaching a peak of over 5 million in 1994, the number of families receiving this assistance fell to just over 2 million by the early 2000s, and remained at that level even after the global financial crisis (Falk, 2016). Reductions were most significant in states that employed the most severe sanctioning policies (Griggs and Evans, 2010), and reflected both *decreased entry to*, and *increased exits from*, 'welfare rolls' (Ray et al., 2014). Between 1995 and 2004, it is estimated that overall TANF participation rates amongst the eligible population fell by half, linked to a combination of families being 'sanctioned off' welfare, failing to meet new eligibility criteria and being dissuaded (rationally) or discouraged (emotionally) from applying in the first place by the programme's stringent conditionality (Parrott and Sherman, 2007; Moffitt, 2008).

Second, however, data linking conditional welfare programmes to positive labour market and poverty reduction outcomes is much weaker. Thus, according to Daguerre (2013), while TANF in the US was regarded 'as a tremendous success on both sides of the political spectrum' (p.4), evidence for its positive effects on job entry is less than compelling, and with respect to earnings/poverty is at best ambiguous and at worse negative (Griggs and Evans, 2010; Ray et al., 2014). While some US studies have identified a link between being sanctioned and entering employment (e.g. Peck, 2007), and some positive impacts on hours worked and earnings (Grogger and Karoly, 2005), others have shown the opposite relationship (e.g. Lee et al., 2004; Wu, 2008), and that for the poorest single parents welfare reform is linked to a further reduction in income (Bavier, 2001). Ray et al. (2014) conclude their review of evidence on US welfare reform by noting that a major part of the 'success' of the reform in terms of reducing welfare caseloads stems from a decline in uptake amongst eligible people, rather than a reduction in the size of the eligible population. This is reflected in an increase in the size of the 'disconnected' population, receiving neither welfare payments nor earnings from work, with inevitable negative consequences for family income and poverty.

UK evidence on the effectiveness of welfare conditionality and sanctions in achieving their ultimate stated goal – getting claimants into sustainable employment – similarly reaches mixed conclusions.

Studies evaluating the impacts of New Labour (1997–2010) activation measures indicate improved employment rates for some of the groups targeted (Ray et al., 2014). The largest rise in employment rates was seen amongst lone parents (McKnight, 2005) and understood to be attributable to a combination of employment support, more generous in-work benefits and conditionality, with the role of earnings-boosting tax credits found to be particularly crucial (Sefton and Sutherland, 2005; Gregg et al., 2006). The conditional 'New Deal for Young People' was also shown to be effective in raising employment levels, but here the wage subsidy was a crucial causal factor, and positive gains appeared to tail off after six years or so, with youth unemployment rates rising from 2004/05 (Ray et al., 2014). The impacts of conditionality targeting sick and disabled benefit claimants during this period are more uncertain, with Ray et al. (2014) describing assessments of programme effectiveness as in the round 'somewhat inconclusive' (p.77). In all these cases, the role of conditionality in achieving programme aims appears to be small, if it exists at all.

There are indications from two UK-based studies (in Northern Ireland) that intensifying job search monitoring can, on its own, reduce registered unemployment levels and the duration of benefit receipt, independent of adjustments in benefit sanctions or other aspects of the conditionality regime (McVicar, 2008, 2010, 2014). Some older UK studies have found that the threat of sanctions was instrumental in persuading some claimants to participate in work programmes (Joyce et al., 2005), or to step up job search activities, especially following a penalty (Peters and Joyce, 2006), but that other claimants were unwilling or unable to comply regardless of the consequences. Comparing the US and UK, Waldfogel (2010) argues that the UK under New Labour was far more successful in reducing poverty precisely because reforms were broader and less employment-focused than in the US. A recent UK National Audit Office report on benefit sanctions reached highly critical conclusions regarding the use of conditionality under the post-2010 Coalition and Conservative administrations, highlighting the absence of compelling UK evidence on employment-related impacts, and whether any such impacts outweigh the costs (see below) of the current regime (National Audit Office, 2016).

Third, most of the available evidence on the impacts of benefit conditionality and sanctions is short- rather than long-term in nature.

For example, European evidence on the short-term effects of actually-imposed sanctions on unemployed benefit claimants demonstrates a consistent and substantial increase in employment entry rates and/or reduced unemployment durations, particularly when sanctions occur early in a claim (Muller and Steiner, 2008; Hofmann, 2008). However, one key study involving longitudinal analysis of administrative data in Switzerland, which considered the effect of both the threat and imposition of sanctions, found that sanctions actually *lowered* the likelihood of sustainable employment and incomes over time (Arni et al., 2009).

Fourth, and highly relevant to the question of the effectiveness of welfare sanctions in 'driving' behavioural change, are the findings from a wide range of studies about claimant knowledge and understanding (Griggs and Evans, 2010; see also Wright and Stewart, 2016). Evidence from both the UK and US indicates that, while welfare recipients are usually aware that penalties are part of the system, they often have little knowledge of when they could be imposed or how they could be avoided or reversed, implying that claimants are often 'effectively being punished for a lack of understanding rather than (deliberate) non-compliance' (Griggs and Evans, 2010, p.6). An independent review of the operation of benefit sanctions in the UK raised particular concerns around the poor understanding of the sanctioning system amongst vulnerable claimants with support needs (Oakley, 2014), and the specific vulnerability of homeless people to sanctions has been well documented (Batty et al., 2015). Lack of understanding amongst claimants was also a key theme to emerge from a large-scale qualitative study of out-of-work benefit claimants in the UK (Dwyer and Bright, 2016; Dwyer et al., 2016; Johnsen et al., 2016; Wright et al., 2016; Wright and Stewart, 2016). It appears that very few make an active choice not to meet the conditions of benefit receipt (Goodwin, 2008; Scottish Government, 2013; Wright and Stewart, 2016), and that in a high proportion of cases sanctions follow vulnerability, lack of understanding, or poor recording of job search, rather than actual 'behavioural flaws'. This was the emphatic conclusion of Reeve's (2017; see also Batty et al., 2015) research with homeless people subject to benefit conditionality in the UK, which found that 'respondents were either set conditions far exceeding their capabilities, or encountered practical and systemic barriers preventing them from complying' (Reeve, 2017, p.73).

Evidence on the effectiveness of conditional and allied approaches in other welfare realms tends to be weak and is, if anything, even more mixed. As discussed in Chapter 4, with respect to street homelessness, for example, Johnsen and Fitzpatrick (2007, 2010) found that, when combined with individually tailored support, sanction-backed 'enforcement' interventions could prompt vulnerable individuals to engage with services, such as substance misuse programmes, which could have 'life saving' results in some instances. But behavioural responses to these sorts of interventions were unpredictable and could instead result in the 'diversion' of vulnerable people into more dangerous activities and places, leading the authors to conclude that they represented a 'high risk strategy' (2007, p.ix). Conditionality targeting tenants of public housing too appears to achieve mixed results. There is compelling evidence on the effectiveness of Family Intervention Projects in tackling anti-social behaviour, which can incorporate housing-focused conditionality via probationary tenancies (see Chapter 4). But evaluations suggest that it is the intensive and multi-faceted support offered through these projects, rather than the use of sanctions, that can help families achieve positive outcomes and address problematic behaviour (Flint, 2011; Batty and Flint, 2012).

Australia has been at the forefront of a number of examples of conditional welfare specifically seeking to promote child welfare, but these have been subject to highly varying degrees of success and controversy. For example, conditionality-backed immunisation initiatives linked to entitlement to family benefits and in place for two decades now are 'generally regarded as successful and as enjoying a broad acceptance throughout Australian society' (Taylor et al., 2016, p.11). The effectiveness of more recent attempts to link family benefits to children's enrolment in school has been less clear. In a performance audit of the programme, the Australian National Audit Office concluded that 'whether [it] has stimulated an increase in underlying enrolment ... is not readily identifiable' (ANAO, 2014, pp.66–67). Taylor et al. (2016) contend that this may reflect a poor programme rationale that does not sufficiently account for the actual (complex and structural) causes of truancy. As discussed in Chapter 4, particular controversy has surrounded Compulsory Income Management policies which have disproportionately impacted on Indigenous Australians. A

large-scale and longitudinal independent evaluation of these measures could find no substantive evidence of the 'program having significant changes relative to its key policy objectives, including changing people's behaviours' (Bray et al., 2014, p.xxi).

Across all forms of conditionality, there is an important distinction to be drawn between the 'threat' of a sanction and the 'imposition' of one, though both can have behavioural impacts (see Chapter 3). Indeed, if policy-makers' priority is to change behaviour (rather than more punitive objectives, see Chapter 6), the most desirable scenario is that 'threat effects' are achieved, with behaviour change secured without the need to impose a sanction (and incur the administrative and wider social costs of doing so; see below). However, evaluations of effectiveness have reached varying conclusions on the potency of 'threat effects' (Griggs and Evans, 2010). In the case of conditionality targeting out-of-work benefit claimants, relevant studies do indicate that the (mere) threat of sanctions positively impacts on job entry, job search and/or compliance with conditions (Lalive et al., 2002; Lee et al., 2004; Joyce et al., 2005; Svarer, 2007; Arni et al., 2009). However, an evaluation of a UK pilot programme testing housing allowance sanctions as a means to discourage anti-social behaviour documents varying responses to the threat of this sanction: 'Some individuals were reported to be very apologetic and to change their behavior, others denied wrong doing and were indignant and in some cases individuals simply did not believe that action would be taken' (Flint et al., 2011, p.23). The issue of 'credibility' was key, as while the penalty – ultimately, eviction – was seen as 'the ultimate sanction' (p.24), some households either did not believe that eviction proceedings would be initiated, or were relatively unconcerned given their confidence that they would easily find alternative accommodation in the private rented sector instead.

There are also wider, but nevertheless intended, impacts of welfare conditionality on societal norms and behaviours. For example, an explicit aim of barring or delaying access to out-of-work benefits to those who 'voluntarily' leave employment is to discourage this behaviour, driven by a policy desire to reinforce the moral 'duty' on people to work if they are able to – a moral duty endorsed by those as diverse as Mead (1986), T. H. Marshall, Lenin and Trotsky (see White, 2003). Thus retrospective welfare conditions can be understood as seeking to promote 'desirable' social behaviours, not just amongst the present cohort of benefit claimants, but also amongst the population as a whole, or at least that portion of the population who recognise that they may in the future require access to welfare benefits. There is no evidence that we are aware of that such measures do in practice have the desired impacts, but the discussion above furnishes a range of reasons to be sceptical, including potential welfare claimants' lack of awareness of these prior conditions (see Peters and Joyce, 2006) and because concerns related to future welfare entitlement may be crowded out by other more immediate considerations.

Another potential wider impact of welfare conditionality, which may or may not be intended, concerns its impact on take-up levels because, as noted above, people may be deterred from accessing welfare support in the first place, or drop out of the system altogether, because of the perceived burden of meeting relevant requirements (Griggs and Evans, 2010). Empirical evidence attests to the effectiveness of this 'hassle-factor' in practice in the US (Moffitt, 2003), where high levels of initial conditionality explicitly aim to 'divert' potential recipients away from making a claim (Rosenberg et al., 2008). The US conservative commentator Lawrence Mead (see Chapter 4) is a strong proponent of the desirability of such 'diversion' tactics, arguing that social security policy should be designed to offer both 'help and hassle' – help into work, and hassle off benefits (Mead, 2005). From his 'new paternalist' perspective, this approach is in the long-term interests of claimants themselves, who are more likely to move into work than they would in the absence of such 'hassle'. Advocates of this model would also take the view that, even if ex-benefit claimants do not move into work, the fact that they are unwilling to subject themselves to the rigour of claiming indicates that they have alternative means of support (e.g. from friends and family) available to them.

Unlike the US, it is not clear in the UK that a large group of lone parents are disconnected from work and welfare (Ray et al., 2014), although there is a growing concern that this may be the case for some other groups, in particular young people (Watts et al., 2014; Loopstra et al., 2015a; National Audit Office, 2016; Devany, 2017). Moreover, explicit political and intellectual support for such 'diversion' has been considerably less strong to date (Finn and Goodship, 2014). This reflects a concern that 'diverted' potential applicants may become isolated from support (including support with finding work), at risk of exploitation or abuse (from family or friends they are forced to rely on), forced into anti-social alternative means of survival (e.g. crime), and/or face severe poverty, including absolute destitution (Fitzpatrick et al., 2016; Geiger, 2012; Devany, 2017). It is to these potentially negative 'spill-over' effects of welfare conditionality, particularly where such effects are unintended, to which we now turn our attention.

## Unintended, spill-over and scar effects

As this review of the effectiveness of conditionality has begun to show, conditional forms of welfare can have a range of unintended impacts. Most well documented on this point is the material hardship experienced by (some) sanctioned benefit claimants, particularly those in low-income groups with dependents and/or no other source of income (e.g. from savings or family/friend/partner support) (Griggs and Evans, 2010). While some critics would argue that the 'punishment' of non-compliers is now an explicit objective of policy (Webster, 2015a), supporters of sanctions would argue that the infliction of suffering is not an intended policy outcome, but rather the aim is to influence claimants' behaviour by incentivising them to actively seek work and move off benefits (Miscampbell, 2014).

However, to say that an outcome is unintended, in the sense that is not actively sought, is not the same as saying that it is unforeseeable. While in the UK case sanctioned claimants are able to apply for a reduced-level 'hardship payment', these awards are discretionary and subject to stringent access rules, with well under half (and historically only one in 10) of sanctioned unemployed claimants actually receiving them (Webster, 2015b). An independent review found that the most vulnerable claimants find it hardest to access hardship payments, in part because 'only those claimants that asked about help in Jobcentre Plus were told about the hardship system' (Oakley, 2014, p.38). The rapid growth in benefit sanctions in the period running up to 2013 (see Chapter 4) has been associated with debt and rent arrears (Wright and Stewart, 2016), homelessness (Reeve, 2017) and large-scale destitution in the UK (Fitzpatrick et al., 2016). The role of sanctions in driving food poverty and growing resort to food banks by low-income people in the UK has now been well established (Sosenko et al., 2013; Loopstra et al., 2015b; Lambie-Mumford, 2017), and sanctioned claimants suffering from diabetes have highlighted the acute challenges this can bring (Wright and Stewart, 2016). In the US, full-family sanctions have been shown to cause food insecurity, serious housing problems, disconnection from electricity and phone connections, and inability to secure necessary medical care (Lindhorst and Mancoske, 2006; see also Griggs and Evans, 2010).

Linked to these material impacts, benefit sanctions and conditionality have also been linked by some authors to negative physical and mental health outcomes, increased stress and reduced emotional wellbeing (Dorsett, 2008; Goodwin, 2008; Peters and Joyce, 2006; Griggs and Evans, 2010). Qualitative research in the UK with a number of groups targeted by welfare conditionality has highlighted that 'extreme anxiety' (Johnsen, 2016, p.7) is, for some individuals, associated not only with being sanctioned (and the associated stress of managing financial hardship and sometimes associated debt), but also more generally with the expectation of attending a relevant appointment in which they may face the risk of sanction (Dwyer and Bright, 2016; Dwyer et al., 2016; Johnsen, 2016; Wright and Stewart, 2016; Wright et al., 2016). In extreme cases, sanctions have been linked to self-harm and suicide attempts (Batty et al., 2015; Wright and Stewart, 2016), something now explicitly recognised by official guidance advising frontline workers how to respond to claimants expressing suicidal intent (Ryan, 2015).

A survey of the impacts of conditionality on a sample of around 1,000 individuals with current or recent experience of homelessness in the UK (Batty et al., 2015) starkly demonstrated the impacts of sanctions on mental health:

> Many sanctioned respondents already suffered problems such as depression, anxiety, stress and panic attacks and some had diagnoses of schizophrenia and bipolar disorder. We know for example that 45 per cent of respondents reporting mental ill health were sanctioned. Many were managing their illnesses effectively. The experience of being sanctioned, however,

> exacerbated these problems, occasionally to the point where respondents could no longer function.
>
> *(p.47)*

This same research also identified a range of other unintended 'spill-over' effects of conditionality targeted at this already vulnerable group, including exacerbating or causing homelessness and putting pressure on relationships with friends and family, who were often financially struggling themselves, as well as undermining attempts to build or maintain relationships with their (often non-resident) children. In these situations, continued reliance on family and friends for support could lead to arguments, friendships turning sour and even relationship breakdown (Batty et al., 2015).

Amongst the most-concerning potential 'spill-over' impacts of conditionality raised by some authors has been the risk of driving people towards acquisitive crime. This has been identified as a 'coping mechanism' for some individuals in response to the hardship associated with being sanctioned in both quantitative and qualitative studies (Machin and Marie, 2004; Griggs and Evans, 2010; Batty et al., 2015; Dwyer and Bright, 2016), in addition to other 'socially undesirable' responses such as begging (Batty et al., 2015). Even more alarmingly, there is some tentative evidence from the US linking severe sanctioning practice to increased levels of child maltreatment (abuse and neglect) (Grogger and Karoly, 2005; Griggs and Evans, 2010). This chimes with a wider evidence base demonstrating a 'strong association between family poverty and a child's chance of suffering child abuse or neglect' (Bywaters et al., 2016, p.ii), as well as between poverty and domestic violence (Fahmy et al., 2016).

Sanctions can also have counter-productive 'scar effects' in generating hostility towards support services and/or more negative views about work (Dorsett, 2008; Joyce et al., 2005). Fletcher (2008), for example, argues that benefit sanctioning may strengthen the hostility of offenders towards forms of authority, propelling them further away from the benefit system and mainstream institutions. This may damage the potential for co-operative or supportive interactions between the sanction giver and receiver, prompting in Ruth Lister's (2004) language a 'getting back at' response to professionals (see also Deacon, 2004), or alternatively resignation to the compliance-based process of 'signing on'. From a behavioural sciences perspective, Bertrand et al. (2004) highlight the likely costs of welfare provision that has an 'adversarial tone, accompanied by monitoring concern, and low expectations', suggesting that 'welfare programs may benefit from triggering more positive attitudes' (p.422). Recent qualitative research with UK jobseekers (Wright et al., 2016) has indicated highly variable experiences of employment support, ranging from individuals describing their adviser as 'a really caring helpful person' (p.7) to other examples where the presence of scarring effects is very clear. Wright et al. (2016) describe 'an impersonal approach ... [which] could create a particular dynamic between Jobcentre Plus advisers and claimants, which some interviewees experienced as intimidating, dehumanising, and disempowering, "just all threats"' (p.6). One job seeker described the process as follows:

> he's not even looking at you ... 'If you don't do that, we'll sanction you. If you don't do that we'll sanction' – everything is a sanction, sanction, sanction, that's all you get ... It's like being bullied, 'If you don't do as I tell you, I'm going to take some money off you.'
>
> *(p.7)*

Evidence of directly counter-productive outcomes of (threatened) sanctions can also be identified in welfare domains other than cash transfer benefits. In housing, for example, removal of security of tenure has been argued to undermine, rather than enhance, work incentives for social tenants in England and Australia (Fitzpatrick and Pawson, 2014; Fitzpatrick and Watts, 2017), and in Australia compulsory income management has been shown to actually *increase* dependence on welfare and erode capabilities, in direct opposition to its aims (Bray et al., 2014). Some would argue that the same applies to certain conditional responses to homelessness and rough sleeping: the No Second Night Out model used in London, which attempts to impose a 'single service offer' on rough sleepers, has been viewed as extremely controversial given its potential to further isolate a highly vulnerable population from support (Johnsen et al., forthcoming).

Reflecting back to Chapter 2's discussion on sanctions and incentives, and their contested interrelationship, leads us to a slightly more abstract concern associated with the potential unintended consequences of these instruments of social control in public policy. Namely that, as a form of 'extrinsic' motivation for those targeted to behave in a particular way, these instruments may crowd out 'intrinsic' motivations, like duty and a sense of obligation, public-spiritedness, of 'doing the right thing, altruism or reciprocity. Moreover, according to Self-Determination Theory, intrinsic motivation is associated not just with better 'performance' against the goal sought, but also with enhanced health and wellbeing, by virtue of meeting people's fundamental psychological needs for competence and autonomy (Deci and Ryan, 2008). This is a key argument put forward by Grant (2012) in her ethical interrogation of incentives, further discussed in Chapter 6. She contends that incentives risk corrupting the character of both the individuals being 'incentivised' and the institutions doing the 'incentivising', with any subsequent removal of the incentive potentially leaving a void in which pro-social behaviour is not sustained by intrinsic motivations that may have existed prior to its introduction (see also Titmuss, 1970/1997).

Finally, there has been much debate about the broader political impacts of the entire discourse around conditional welfare. Fletcher et al. (2016) have argued that 'a principle of conditionality in welfare and the need to protect against the cynical manipulation of gaming the welfare system is a pervasive, if not hegemonic, idea supported by welfare practitioners and recipients [in the UK]' (p.183). Friedli and Stearn (2015) similarly argue that 'The discourse of "psychological deficit" has become an established feature of the UK policy literature on unemployment and social security' (p.40, and see Chapter 3), echoing Watson's claim that 'the very discourse of conditionality recasts what are in essence structural economic problems as the project of a deficient work ethic among individuals' (2015, p.651). Far from conditionality ensuring the support of the wider public for welfare programmes (see Chapter 1), some have argued that it does precisely the opposite by promoting an individualised and stigmatising discourse, and supporting a 'politics of resentment' (Hoggett et al., 2013). Drawing on Grover (2010), Hoggett argues that:

> framing policies to appease real or imagined resentments strengthens, rather than mollifies, the underlying sense of grievance. This in turn can potentially lead to a perverse cycle of increasingly vindictive forms of welfare conditionality. Language, and particularly political language, has a performative dimension to it and can create what it purports to describe.
>
> *(p.16)*

Such perspectives parallel debates in criminal justice regarding the interrelationship between public opinion and penal policy (Frost, 2010), and raise the important question of the origins of public support for welfare conditionality and harsh sanctioning policies. Recent analysis of the British Social Attitudes survey has highlighted that 'top down' influences are extremely important in driving negative public attitudes towards benefit claimants and declining public support for the benefits system (O'Grady, 2017).

## Costs

Even where it can be demonstrated that a particular conditional welfare programme achieves its intended aims, with zero or minimal unintended impacts, the question remains whether it is a cost-efficient means of achieving these ends. Thus, of core relevance to assessing the overall impacts of conditionality are the costs, both financial and non-financial, of implementing it.

The implementation of conditional welfare, and specifically the monitoring and verification processes that are an indispensable feature of conditional programmes (see Chapter 2), come with a financial cost in terms of administrative infrastructure and staff time (Bastagli, 2009; Fiszbein et al., 2009), albeit that these costs will vary depending on the intensity, frequency and extent of the surveillance undertaken.

The costs of monitoring and verification have been estimated for CCTs programmes in three Latin American countries, which suggest they can vary as widely as between 2% and 24% of total programme costs (Caldés et al., 2006). Another study of 10 CCT programmes estimated overall administrative costs of 4–10% of total programme resources, with monitoring compliance specifically estimated to absorb 1–3% of total costs (Grosh et al., 2008). In social housing, the bureaucratic costs of administering multiple fixed-term tenancy regimes, and 'pay to stay' policies, have been considered prohibitive, and to potentially heavily outweigh any gains in terms of increased rental revenues (Fitzpatrick and Watts, 2017). In other programmes, the costs of implementation may be far less daunting, for instance, where school attendance can be monitored automatically through school records, or vaccinations through already collected health records (Fiszbein et al., 2009).

There are also costs to claimants or recipients, both in terms of time spent demonstrating compliance (e.g. travelling to and from appointments or mandatory training and collecting required documentation), and sometimes in financial terms too. Evaluations of CCTs, for example, have highlighted the sometimes very high financial costs associated with compliance. In the case of one programme, the time spent demonstrating compliance was estimated to amount to the equivalent of almost half of the value of the cash transfer (Pellerano and Barca, 2014). Where CCTs seek to promote children's school attendance, families will likely weigh the costs of complying with the income foregone by children not taking part in paid work. Where these costs outweigh the value of the transfer, programme aims are unlikely to be achieved (Fiszbein et al., 2009).

It must also be borne in mind that meeting behavioural requirements to demonstrate compliance with conditional regimes is not necessarily coterminous with achieving the ultimate behavioural aims sought. Those targeted might seek to *demonstrate* compliance without actually complying (Fletcher et al., 2016), or may in all good faith go to great efforts to comply but in ways that do not in fact achieve the intended aims of the policy. For example, claimants of Universal Credit in the UK can be required to participate in job search activities for up to 35 hours a week, and have reported that doing so has in fact

> prevented them from pursuing more meaningful approaches to improving employability, such as volunteering or work trials, which could serve to enhance experience, learn skills, build confidence and develop networks that could lead to suitable and sustainable job outcomes.
>
> *(Wright et al., 2016, p.5)*

Batty et al. (2015) recorded similar 'perverse outcomes' in their study of impacts of conditionality on those experiencing homelessness, with another study finding that frontline workers in homelessness services in the UK view the current conditionality regime 'as a box-ticking exercise which takes insufficient account of individual circumstances and does little to enhance this group's prospects of employment' (Johnsen et al., 2016, p.8).

It is thus not only the time and effort of the recipient that can be wastefully expended, but support and advocacy services can also find significant resources absorbed by efforts to help clients challenge the negative outcomes of such processes. In the UK, single and youth homelessness services have reported the major knock-on effects of the sanctions regime, in terms of staff time required to support their clients in meeting work-related requirements and challenging 'adverse decisions' (Fitzpatrick et al., 2015), at the direct expense of time spent helping them access settled accommodation or tackle addiction issues (Johnsen et al., 2016). Other studies have highlighted the short-sightedness of the 'valorisation of work' (Patrick, 2012, p.11) to the exclusion of a wide range of other activities with substantial social and community benefits, including parenting, care work, volunteering and advocacy.

There are less tangible costs too, with higher levels of 'judgment and intrusion into a client's personal life' required to assess whether claimants meet behavioural requirements than those required to assess other kinds of eligibility criteria or thresholds of need (Watson, 2015, p.648). At a societal level, the value accorded to privacy and freedom will therefore need to be weighed in the balance against the behavioural benefits sought via conditional welfare (Flint and Nixon, 2006; Flint, 2006). Privacy-related concerns lie at the core of Pérez-Muñoz's (2017) argument against the compulsory drug testing of welfare recipients in the US. Conceptualising drug testing as an intrusive privacy violation, Pérez-Muñoz (2017) argues that a very strong empirical case for the benefits of such an approach – vis-à-vis 'promoting welfare recipients' self-sufficiency and responsibility or [avoiding] harm to third parties' – would be required to morally defend such an approach (p.13, and see also Chapter 6). His review of 'current empirical realities' (p.10) – including highly unequal 'background conditions' influencing who experiences addiction issues, the absence of any link between drug testing and 'feasible opportunities for rehabilitation' (p.12), and evidence that 'tends to support the view that drug testing produces more harm than it prevents' (p.13) – leads him to conclude that 'drug testing for welfare recipients by itself is an insufficient and morally impermissible instrument for achieving ... desired goals' (p.13).

Thus, where there are demonstrated gains in relation to, for instance, labour market participation or health care utilisation from the conditionality embedded in welfare programmes, these must set against not only the direct costs of administering welfare programmes on a conditional basis, but also the documented additional costs to the welfare service user themselves and wider society of this model. Only by considering these gains and losses in the round, including any relevant trade-offs and cost offsets, is it possible to come to a firm view on the full impact (intended and unintended, positive or negative) of behaviourally conditional forms of welfare. The ethical implications of these considerations are the focus of the next chapter. But first we consider whether there might be (more attractive) alternative routes to relevant behaviour-change goals than welfare conditionality.

## Alternatives

As noted in Chapter 1, welfare conditionality is at root a method of social control, a means of exerting power over people. However, there are a variety of alternative means of exerting power over targeted populations and inducing them to alter their behaviour in ways desired by public policy. Given that we have established above that welfare conditionality can be a costly and uncertain means of achieving desired forms of behavioural change, and can carry negative unintended consequences, it is natural to consider the efficacy of other methods to reach conduct-shaping objectives (the ethics or otherwise of both these objectives, and the methods employed to achieve them, are considered in the next chapter).

Drawing on Bachrach and Baratz (1963), Lukes (2005) and Grant (2006), we have developed a typology of social control interventions (Watts et al., 2017; Johnsen et al., forthcoming). This distinguishes between: '*force*', wherein compliance is secured via the removal of the possibility of choosing not to comply (e.g. arresting or imprisoning people as well as physical forms of punishment or restraint); '*coercion*', where compliance is ensured via the threat of deprivation (benefit sanctions would be the archetypal form); '*bargaining*', which incentivises behaviour via the exchange of gains and losses (incentive-based CCT programmes could be thought of in this way); and '*influence*', where compliance is sought via persuasive efforts to shape people's beliefs, judgements or behaviour (for example, forms of assertive outreach that seek to persuade rough sleepers to engage with support and 'come inside').

Probably the best known, and possibly most controversial, example of this final 'influencing' category are 'nudge' interventions, associated with the authors Thaler and Sunstein (2008) and now a prominent behaviour-change technique that has gained public-sector backing in the UK, US and Australia and earned Richard Thaler the 2017 Nobel Prize for Economics. Drawing on insights from behavioural economics, 'nudges' seek to steer people towards decisions and behaviours that benefit themselves and society. They do so by altering the framing of a decision (the 'choice architecture') in order to encourage (though not enforce) 'good choices'. This 'nudge' approach is argued to be paternalistic because it seeks to influence people's behaviour in order to encourage them to live longer, healthier, more productive lives. It is also presented as libertarian in the sense that 'choices are not blocked, fenced off, or significantly burdened' (2008, p.5). Despite their 'non-conditional' nature, nudge techniques have been subject to fierce criticism on the basis that they are manipulative and undemocratic and promote 'shallow' and unsustainable forms of behaviour change (Goodwin, 2012, p.91; see also John et al., 2009; Marteau et al., 2011). Defenders of nudges counter that 'there is no such thing as "neutral" design' (Thaler and Sunstein, 2008, p.3), with market forces continually manipulating consumer preferences and actions via self-serving nudges, and argue that it is therefore legitimate – even necessary – for governments to employ 'counter-nudges' to influence people's behaviour in the pursuit of societal goals (Oliver, 2013; Curchin, 2017). An emphasis on deliberative, democratic and transparent decision making regarding the aims and uses of 'nudge techniques' has been advocated as a means to address some of these concerns, while retaining 'nudges' as a policy tool (Hausman and Welch, 2010; Jones et al., 2013).

In addition to the plethora of options provided by 'nudge-like' techniques, policy-makers also have at their disposal other non-forceful and non-coercive means of pursuing behavioural change objectives, key amongst them measures seeking to influence behaviour via the provision of information. Singer (2015), for instance, highlights the findings of a comparative study of the cost effectiveness of interventions seeking to increase the time children spend in schools in developing countries, including CCTs and UCTs but also scholarships, free school uniforms, health-related programmes and the provision of information to parents about the increased future wages of those who stay in school. The study found that by far the most cost-effective intervention was information provision, achieving substantially greater impacts on school attendance than cash transfers (conditional or not) (Dhaliwal et al., 2014).

Also relevant are the more informal modes of influence at the disposal of 'street-level bureaucrats' in their face-to-face interactions with those using welfare supports, including praise/blame, approval/disapproval, and stigma/acceptance (Chriss, 2007). It has indeed been argued that the perceived failure of 'self-governing' citizens and communities to regulate themselves through informal mechanisms of social and self-control has led to the 'return of the state' and the 're-emergence of vertical state–citizen relationships' (Flint, 2002, p.259; see also Chriss, 2007), of which conditionality is just one example.

This discussion serves to highlight that in securing behaviour change, those implementing welfare programmes can make use of a wide range of formal and informal, 'hard' and 'soft' social control mechanisms, quite aside from explicit conditionality and sanctioning, to steer behaviour. The effectiveness of conditionality will in practice depend on how these formal and informal mechanisms come together in specific programmes and contexts. The role of 'street-level bureaucrat' discretion is of course key – as a vast literature from Lipsky (1980/2010) onwards demonstrates – but that is not the same as saying that programme structure and design do not matter. These factors frame, shape and define the parameters of how policies can be implemented in highly significant ways (Pellerano and Barca, 2014; Watts, 2014). Indeed, Pellerano and Barca (2014), in their review of the design of CCTs, argue that behaviour can be 'conditioned' in at least four different ways, only one of which involves 'explicit conditionality'. Others include how a programme is labelled (which will give behavioural signals, e.g. 'child benefit' in the UK), how it is delivered (e.g. to a mother or a father, in cash or in kind), or the provision of information or training alongside welfare provision.

The key point here is that explicit behavioural conditionality, whether in its coercive or bargaining form, is not the only tool in welfare policy-makers' chests. Nevertheless, it remains clear that conduct conditionality remains the central and dominant framing of much welfare policy pursuing a behaviour-change agenda in many countries, hence the central focus of this book. This raises the question, then, why sanctions are the dominant conduct-steering technique employed in relation to welfare service users, while more subtle and diverse techniques are employed to achieve other forms of behaviour change targeting wider groups of the population.

Even leaving to one side for now the fundamental challenge laid to this entire behaviour-change agenda by evidence on the structural causes of unemployment (see Chapter 1), this focus on coercive-conditionality is especially significant because of the comparatively much greater impacts on low-income groups of the associated sanctions than the minor (or non-existent) sanctions associated with milder forms of social control. Compare, for instance, the token charge imposed for not bringing a bag of one's own to the supermarket, or the cost of driving into the central London congestion zone, to the impact of being late to a Jobcentre appointment or failing to seek work actively enough (the withdrawal of all or a substantial proportion of unemployment benefit for a period of weeks, months or even years) or failing to meet the behavioural conditions attached to a tenancy (eviction). The ethical import of these distributional questions is clear, and again picked up in the next chapter.

## Concluding comments

This chapter has demonstrated the complex questions posed by the apparently straightforward empirical matter of whether conditionality 'works' in bringing about desired forms of behaviour change. Many, especially from the political Left, have challenged this proposition by ridiculing the 'rational economic man' model of human action said to underpin welfare conditionality. We have argued that criticisms based on attacking the literal 'truth' of perfect rationality are wide of the mark, and often rest on a misrepresentation of much of the literature employing these models. It remains entirely reasonable – and indeed helpful – to assume in many if not most cases at least a 'thin' level of highly contextualised rationality of welfare recipients, while taking into account the numerous and well-evidenced insights of the behavioural sciences. Indeed, an appreciation of such 'utility maximising' (or loss-avoiding) responses on the part of those subject to conditional forms of welfare is key to understanding why conditionality is in practice ineffective in some circumstances, for instance, when the 'real' cost of compliance exceeds the burden of the sanction. Nonetheless, critiques of the rational actor theory do serve to usefully highlight that the impacts of conditionality will vary substantially by context, and even by individual, something clearly borne out in evidence about its effectiveness.

Empirical evidence on the impacts and outcomes of welfare conditionality is extremely mixed in its conclusions, not only in relation to its efficacy as a technique in achieving programme goals, but also the wider implications of its deployment for both welfare service users and broader society. For CCTs in developing-country contexts there is a rich seam of evidence, so too to some extent for the widespread use of behavioural conditions and sanctions in developed welfare states. The findings of these two strands of evidence are far from conclusive, with consensus on the effectiveness of these different kinds of conditionality still elusive. What is beyond doubt is that some CCT programmes do achieve programme objectives, reducing poverty and promoting engagement with education or health provision. What is less clear is whether the conditionality of CCTs is core to achieving these positive outcomes, or whether non-conditional approaches ('unconditional' cash transfers or even the better provision of information and education) would be equally as effective. Equally, the capacity of conditional benefits in advanced welfare contexts to 'hassle' many recipients out of the benefit system is not in doubt, but the longer-term gains, in terms of sustained entries into employment and of poverty, are far less clear.

There is at the same time considerable evidence of financial hardship and material deprivation imposed by sanctions on some welfare recipients, particularly those who are most vulnerable, as well as significant impacts on mental and physical health, and some suggestion of 'scarring effects' that damage relationships between service providers and service users. There are in addition a range of far from insignificant costs associated with welfare conditionality, for both the administrative system and service users themselves. Extremely concerning, but supported to date by only limited and indirect evidence, are links between sanctioning and higher rates of crime and child maltreatment.

Evaluations of conditional programmes in welfare realms beyond cash transfers also reach mixed conclusions. While conditional interventions seeking to compel rough sleepers to engage with some support have been cited as 'saving lives' in some cases, in others they have been shown to drive highly vulnerable people into even more dangerous situations. While Australia's use of conditionality to drive immunisation rates appears to have been a relatively uncontroversial success, attempts in parts of Australia and the UK to use fixed-term tenancies to drive behaviour change appear to have been an unmitigated failure to date.

Given the complexities and shortcomings of welfare conditionality as a behaviour-change tool, we also explored alternative 'social control' mechanisms, including 'nudges' and other influencing techniques, highlighting that 'hard' sanctions are far from being the only tool in the welfare policy-makers' chests. This in turn prompted reflection on why sanctions in particular were apparently most commonly deployed in systems focused on the poorest groups in society, particularly given their acknowledged harsh consequences in many instances. This and other matters pertaining to the 'consequences' of welfare conditionality lie at the heart of its ethical defensibility, or otherwise, as examined in the next chapter.

# 6

# THE ETHICS OF CONDITIONALITY

It will be clear by now that welfare conditionality as a whole, particularly in its more 'behavioural' guises, raises a host of profound moral questions and dilemmas. This chapter seeks to interrogate these dilemmas and in so doing provide a framework for systematic ethical analysis and assessment. It explores how welfare conditionality can be understood and evaluated using a range of normative frameworks, i.e. frameworks that explicitly engage in questions of values, morals and ethics.[1] Drawn largely from moral and political philosophy, these normative frameworks offer different (sometimes overlapping, at other times competing) answers to the question 'how should society – and the relationship between citizens and the state – be organised?'

We begin by considering what it is about welfare conditionality that makes it so often seem ethically troubling, taking as our 'stepping off' point Ruth Grant's (2012) formative work on the ethical legitimacy of the use of incentives in public policy (and other spheres) to change behaviour (see Chapter 3). We go on to consider the moral case for and against the diverse forms of welfare conditionality, as viewed via a series of philosophically-informed normative 'lenses', including rights-based, utilitarian, contractualist, communitarian, paternalist and social justice perspectives. The continuities and discontinuities between these ethical perspectives, and the potential for reconciling them, at least in certain contexts, will be explored over the course of the chapter and picked up again in Chapter 7.

## Conditionality as an ethical 'problem'

As explained in the introduction, behavioural forms of welfare conditionality are, at heart, forms of social control – exercises of *power over* claimants and recipients of publicly-funded welfare programmes. More specifically, conditionality is a form of *coercive* power (Lukes, 2005) which uses the threat of deprivation of welfare goods (rather than force, bargaining or persuasion) to achieve behavioural change on the part of those in seeking access to these goods (Watts et al., 2017; Johnsen et al., 2018).

As such, behavioural conditionality seems, on the face of it, to require robust ethical justification because of the challenge that it poses both to notions of liberty, given its coercive quality, and also to egalitarian notions of justice, because of the disproportionate (sometimes exclusive) impact on the least well-off in society. Throw into the mix the demonstrable (and in some cases extreme) hardship and deprivation linked to harsher forms of conditionality – most notably full-family sanctions in the US – and fundamental humanitarian objections may arise as well. As Falk et al. (2014) comment:

> [Benefit] Sanctioning represents one of the most difficult conundrums in social policy—families receive aid precisely because they cannot otherwise meet basic needs, yet reducing or ending that aid is the available way in which policymakers can enforce program[me] requirements.
>
> *(p.25)*

Likewise, conditional welfare approaches in developing-world contexts have been described as 'pernicious, atrocious and abominable' by Freeland (2007, p.75) because they operate on the principle that depriving some of the world's poorest people from assistance that they require to meet basic subsistence needs is a legitimate means to some broader ends.

However, over the course of this book we have sought to demonstrate the enormous diversity in welfare interventions that have a behaviourally 'conditional' element. We have shown that they operate in very different ways, are driven by a variety of motives, have widely varying designs, target diverse populations and have distinctive outcomes (both intended and unintended). It is therefore unlikely, even implausible, that a 'universal' conclusion about the ethical legitimacy (or not) of welfare conditionality can be reached. Instead, a more pluralistic and flexible framework is required to assess each form of conditionality on its own merits, and from the perspective of a range of moral standpoints, in order to facilitate normative analysis which is *context-specific, evidence-informed* and *ethically-literate* (see also Geiger, 2017).

Ruth Grant (2002, 2006, 2012) takes precisely this sort of approach in her 'untangling' of the ethical legitimacy of incentives, and this work has much to offer normative consideration of other forms of conditional welfare interventions (see Chapter 3; also Watts et al., 2017). Grant's main objective is to establish that, contrary to the prevailing view in much economics literature, incentives do not necessarily allow for a 'voluntary response' (like other acts of 'power over' other people, they can be manipulative or coercive depending on their specific characteristics). Moreover, whether someone is able to respond voluntarily to such an act of power is not the sole criterion for judging its legitimacy. By conceptualising incentives in this way Grant illuminates a range of ethical questions requiring systematic examination, many of which are equally relevant to sanctions-backed conditionality. Amongst the relevant factors she considers are the effect that the use of incentives – and by extension other modes of social control – have on the 'character' of all of those involved:

> Power relationships can have an impact on the character of all of the individuals involved in any particular interaction: both those who are engaged in making an offer, persuading, or threatening force and those who are responding to offers, argument or threats. *(2012, p.52)*

Impacts on the 'institutional culture' of service provider organisations involved in the delivery of conditional welfare interventions might therefore be one relevant ethical consideration (Gregory, 2015). There has, for example, been significant controversy over the role of those homelessness organisations which have worked with enforcement agents, like the police or border agencies, to address some aspects of street homelessness (see Chapter 4). The argument has been made by some academics and other commentators that these organisations risk becoming simply a 'tool' or 'arm' of government (Buckingham, 2011), losing sight of their fundamental ethos, values and need for independence (see Greer and Horst, 2014; Milbourne and Cushman, 2015), though this has been hotly disputed by some of those directly involved (Swain, 2003, 2015; see also Watts et al., 2017; Johnsen et al., 2018). A converse argument could in any case be made that requirements attached to funding allocated via elected (local or national) governments lend, at least in principle, an important element of democratic legitimacy to the disbursement of public funds. The subversion of these principles by private charitable organisations which accept public money, but are resistant to the 'strings' attached to it, may then present an ethical concern of a different order.

Grant's framework equally requires attention to the impact of welfare conditionality on the character of the welfare recipients targeted. She argues (2006) that 'it makes an ethical difference, both for individual character and for social norms, whether people are motivated by fear of punishment, desire for reward, generosity, or rectitude, and so forth' (p.33). Germane here are the emerging concerns discussed in Chapter 5 that conditional welfare shifts the tenor of relationships between those in receipt of welfare support and frontline workers in highly undesirable ways, 'scarring' the potential role of these relationships in bringing about positive outcomes. Relationships structured by the implementation of conditionality may become fractious, stressful and adversarial; experienced as 'intimidating, dehumanising and disempowering' (Dwyer and Bright, 2016, pp.4–5) and reinforce feelings of stigma and shame that correlate to a wide range of negative social consequences (Phelan et al., 1997; Lister, 2004).

This sits alongside evidence suggesting that personalised, one-to-one, flexible and consistent relationships between frontline workers and those in need of support can play a transformative role in addressing even the complex needs of highly vulnerable individuals (Batty et al.,

2015; Dwyer and Bright, 2016; Fitzpatrick and Watts, 2016). Also relevant here is Grant's argument that 'rational persuasion' 'might be considered *the* morally exemplary form of power' (2006, p.33, emphasis in original) in that it is consistent with 'self-government', something surely more likely to be fostered in the context of supportive relationships too. As well as being 'morally exemplary' for this reason, 'intrinsic motivation' (doing something because one wants to, rather than because one is being incentivised, coerced or forced to) fosters well-being, by virtue meeting people's psychological need for competence and autonomy (Deci and Ryan, 2008, and see Chapter 5).

However, perhaps of most central relevance to our purposes in untangling the ethics of welfare conditionality is Grant's exploration of what counts as a 'legitimate purpose' in the exercise of power. In her view, without such a legitimate purpose, no exercise of power, certainly not of a coercive variety, can be considered ethical. As made clear in Chapter 4, the motives driving different manifestations of conditionality vary immensely. Focusing on benefit sanctions – the archetypal form of conditionality – many critics perceive clear and unacceptable 'punitive intent', viewing them as deliberately disciplinary policies, underpinned by a motivation to 'punish the poor', holding them to standards of conduct not required of more advantaged groups (Dwyer, 1998; Deacon, 2004; Standing, 2011; Fletcher et al., 2016).

Evidence to support this position may be garnered from the fact that the many public welfare 'benefits' enjoyed by better-off sections of the population, certainly in the UK, such as free healthcare at the point of use, subsidised loans for university education, tax relief on home ownership, and so on (Titmuss, 1958; Dwyer, 2010), are seldom accompanied by the sort of rigorous surveillance and behavioural requirements that are applied to the means-tested benefits focused on people living in poverty (Flint, 2002; Standing, 2011). It is this apparent affront to equity and equal treatment that troubles so many critics of welfare conditionality, alongside the unnecessary hardship that they perceive these policies to generate.

Webster (2015a) has gone so far as to argue that the benefit sanctions regime in the UK amounts to a 'secret penal system' which lacks the procedural safeguards associated with the mainstream judicial system (see also Adler, 2016). He also points out that it exacts penalties that are often much harsher (complete cessation of income, sometimes for substantial periods of time) than those applied by the criminal justice system for minor offences. Others, too, have drawn parallels with criminal justice policy, specifically with the 'purposes' of retribution and/or restitution, as well as deterrence, querying whether this is appropriate in a system that is meant to be designed to protect people's welfare (Fletcher, 2013; Fletcher et al., 2016; Fletcher and Wright, 2017).

However, as you would expect, supporters of welfare conditionality mount a number of passionate moral defences of these policies (Mead, 1997; Miscampbell, 2014), as considered in the remainder of this chapter, and the debates play out somewhat differently in developing-world contexts where the aims of welfare conditionality are less easy to characterise as punitive in nature (Bastagli, 2009). Some social policy scholars have also given serious consideration to the potential ethical justifications for conditional welfare interventions. Most notable in the latter camp is Alan Deacon, who in 2004 published an influential paper which placed an analysis of the then Labour government's controversial policies on anti-social behaviour in the context of the broader debate about conditionality in welfare. Deacon (2004) gave detailed attention to three potential justifications for welfare conditionality – contractualist, mutualist, and paternalist justifications – and we examine each of these below in the light of developments described in the preceding chapters. We begin, however, by reviewing the principal normative and discursive lens through which objections to conditionality are most often discussed – that of 'rights' – and what is often viewed as its main rival: 'utilitarianism'.

## Rights

The moral case made against welfare conditionality tends to be rooted in a rights-based vision of a common humanity or social citizenship that is unconditional, at least with respect to the meeting of fundamental needs. Within moral philosophy, the notion of rights has its origins in the Kantian 'deontological' school of thought, which assesses the rightness or wrongness of particular courses of action in terms of the 'universalisable' or 'categorical' duties people owe to each other. Rights can be understood as 'side constraints' (Dworkin, 1977) that (ethically) limit the actions that can be taken in order to pursue collective goals (Kymlicka, 2002). In other words, and in Kant's famous formulation, people must be treated as ends in themselves, not means to other people's ends.

Over the course of several centuries, with an acceleration in the post-war years, the idea of universal 'human rights' has become the dominant normative lens through which progressive social causes – national and international, local and global – are often pursued (Dean, 2004; Woodiwiss, 2005; Lukes, 2008). Such rights are argued to be owed to *all* people on the basis of our common humanity (Turner, 1993). Intrinsic to most human rights discourses (and inherited from the Lockean conception of 'natural rights') is the idea that the 'fundamental' rights they encompass are self-evident, inalienable, and non-negotiable: 'absolute' in other words. Human rights are most often articulated in international instruments and agreements, many of which encompass 'positive' social rights to various forms of welfare. For example, Article 25 of the United Nations Universal Declaration of Human Rights (1948) asserts:

> Everyone has the right to a standard of living adequate for the health and wellbeing of himself and his family, including food, clothing, housing and medical care and necessary social services.

Citizenship rights focus us on the national rather than global realm (Marshall, 1950), but according to some schools of thought should, like human rights, be understood as moral rights that are 'universal', in the sense of applying to all citizens on an unconditional basis (Titmuss, 1968; Townsend, 1979; Dwyer, 2010). In many countries, though not the UK, citizenship rights are codified in written constitutions but are generally unenforceable by the individual citizen. In other words, they are 'political markers of concern' (Bengtsson, 2001, p.255) which 'express goals which political actors ... agree to pursue' (Mabbett, 2005, p.98), rather than instruments that serve to further 'the legal protection of individuals' (Kenna and Uhry, 2006, p.1). As such, they are of a fundamentally different order to the 'black letter' legal entitlements that have occupied much of this book, and with which we contrasted discretionary forms of welfare in Chapter 2.

Regardless of their legal standing, both human and citizenship rights can be viewed as primarily *moral* statements, bringing ethical pressure to bear on relevant states to take measures to change their policy and practice (UNDP, 2000). Conditionality in the provision of core welfare services is often viewed as a logical anathema in this type of rights-based thinking: if people have an absolute moral right to something (e.g. to a basic level of income) then making access to it dependent on conformity to behavioural requirements is unacceptable, given that those who do not meet these requirements will as a consequence have their 'inalienable' rights violated. Moreover, as these rights are 'trumps' (Dworkin, 1977), they cannot be 'traded' against collective gains for the rest of society, such as higher levels of economic productivity, or even for gains (such as increased opportunities to escape poverty) that may at least arguably accrue to the welfare recipient themselves. It is clear, then, that these sorts of human and citizenship rights-based perspectives leave little space for any form of welfare conditionality to be considered morally justifiable.

However, while such 'rights-talk' carries with it considerable ethical and intuitive force, it also poses a number of formidable conceptual and empirical challenges that require some reflection (see also Fitzpatrick et al., 2014).

First, unless one happens to be persuaded by theological arguments, then the question of the philosophical *foundation* of global human rights must be confronted (Turner, 1993). Some have argued that these rights should be understood as 'socially constructed' (Dean, 2004) rather than 'natural' in origin, rooted in universal shared norms about what people should have access to in order to achieve a basic standard of living (for example, Nussbaum, 2000) or to have their basic 'needs' met (Doyal and Gough, 1991; Norman, 1998). However, it is far from clear that such a global 'overlapping consensus' in ethics in fact exists (Finch, 1979; Miller, 1999), with large-scale empirical work undertaken by moral psychologists working within the 'Moral Foundations Theory' tradition demonstrating the 'breadth and variability of the moral domain' across world regions (Graham et al., 2011, p.380). Haidt and Graham (2007), for example, identify five moral foundations in total: Harm/Care, Fairness/Reciprocity, Ingroup/Loyalty, Authority/Respect, and Purity/Sanctity. Crucially, these authors find that this broader conception of morality, which extends well beyond individual-based considerations such as rights and justice (generally bracketed as part of the Fairness/Reciprocity domain) or needs (within the Harm/Care domains), is reflected not just outside but also *within* Western nations. Specifically, those on the political Right-of-centre in Western democracies place 'greater emphasis on concerns about ingroup loyalty, respect for authorities and traditions, and physical/spiritual purity' than those on the Left (Graham et al., 2011, p.380).

Second, the moral 'rights' expressed in international human rights instruments and, very often, in national constitutions too, are almost inevitably *broad and abstract in nature*, in sharp contrast to the detailed and delimited 'black letter' legislative entitlements to welfare referenced above. This means that, on those occasions where such abstract rights do become enforceable via courts (international or domestic), they mark a substantial transfer of policy-making power from the political to the legal sphere. Particularly in the case of social rights such as the rights to welfare provision and support, the granting of wide-ranging policy discretion to the courts implies judges determining the allocation of scarce resources in situations where 'hard choices' have to be made between a range of needy and/or deserving cases (see also King, 2003). The term 'juristocracy' is sometimes used in legal scholarship to indicate circumstances wherein the 'constitutionalisation' of rights has transferred significant amounts of power from representative institutions to judiciaries (see Hirschl, 2007). Such arrangements raise obvious democratic concerns about judges, rather than elected politicians, setting policy aims and resource priorities (Campbell et al., 2011).

Third, and relatedly, it is evidently the case that a number of so-called 'inalienable' moral rights can, and often do, conflict with each other (Waldron, 1993), and the broader and more expansive such rights are, the greater the likelihood of clashes. As Michael Ignatieff (2000) has commented:

> Activists who suppose that the Universal Declaration of Human Rights is a comprehensive list of all the desirable ends of human life fail to understand that these ends – liberty and equality, freedom and security, private property and distributive justice – conflict and, because they do, the rights that define them as

> entitlements are also in conflict ... The idea of rights as trumps implies that when rights are introduced into a political discussion, they serve to resolve the discussion. In fact, the opposite is the case. When political demands are turned into rights claims, there is a real risk that the issue at stake will become irreconcilable, since calling a claim a right is to call it non-negotiable, at least in popular parlance.
>
> *(pp.299–300)*

For all their philosophical and practical limitations, however, human rights frameworks have been argued to constitute a valuable 'discursive resource' (Dean, 2010, p.9) or 'shared vocabulary' (Ignatieff, 2000, p.349) which can help to mobilize collective action aimed at progressive policy reform (Fortman, 2006; Waldron, 1993). Even for some sceptics, the notion of human rights then may be considered a 'useful fiction', justified, perhaps ironically, on the consequentialist basis that they do more good than harm, especially in countries where democratic traditions and the protection of minorities remain weak or underdeveloped (Fitzpatrick et al., 2014).

In developed welfare states too, the incorporation of aspects of human rights frameworks into domestic law can provide a basis for challenging regressive policy developments. In the UK, for example, Human Rights Act 1998-based litigation has successfully challenged the imposition of the so-called 'Bedroom Tax' on certain disabled households (Meers, 2017). However, it is worth bearing in mind that the same human rights-based protection of 'privacy' and 'family life' could make it difficult to abolish private or religiously-segregated education, should a radically-minded government ever wish to do so. Human rights-based frameworks can be deployed for reactionary ends as well as for more progressive ones (Campbell et al., 2011).

The key point here, however, is that, despite its resonance and contemporary dominance, and the fact that one might very often agree with the substantive conclusions reached by 'rights enthusiasts' (e.g. King, 2012), the concept of human rights, and its citizenship variant, is only one normative lens through which to consider the ethical legitimacy (or otherwise) of welfare conditionality. It is also a normative lens that has some significant shortcomings and, crucially, fails to capture the moral concerns and intuitions of substantial sections of the population in even advanced democratic societies (Graham et al., 2011). We would argue, therefore, that a less absolutist, more pluralist (Berlin, 1969) approach to the ethical evaluation of conditionality is required to achieve sustainable political change.

## Utilitarianism

Utilitarianism is the best-known strand within the 'consequentialist' school of moral philosophy which avers, in contradistinction to the deontological rights-based theories just discussed, that the morally best course of action is that which brings about the most desirable or 'valuable' state of affairs. For utilitarians, this valuable state of affairs comprises the maximisation of human 'utility' or 'welfare' – 'the greatest happiness of the greatest number' in Jeremy Bentham's famous formulation. In modern political philosophy, 'utility' is often defined not as a psychic state of mind (happiness) but as (informed) preference-satisfaction, though some utilitarians have focused on other key sources of value, including pleasure, desire, self-interest and well-being (Goodin, 1993). Some have sought instead to put the emphasis on minimising pain, suffering and unhappiness, so-called 'negative utilitarianism' (Smart and Williams, 1973).

As a moral code, utilitarianism has a strong intuitive appeal and has been hugely influential in welfare economics and in other public policy spheres across the Western world. Indeed, Kymlicka (2002) comments that 'in our society utilitarianism operates as a kind of tacit background against which other theories have to assert and defend themselves' (p.10; see also Rawls, 1971/1999). Utilitarianism requires 'equal weight' to be given to each person's interests (Kymlicka, 2002), with the concept of 'declining marginal utility' (that a person will derive less utility from the second unit of a good than from the first) also serving to reinforce this egalitarian dimension, by weighting more heavily the gains (and losses) of those who have least (Goodin, 1993; Gabriel, 2017). The idea that 'urgent claims should be met first' can be understood as a basic component of utilitarian morality (Gabriel, 2017, p.460).

However, intense criticism has focused on the aggregative nature of utilitarianism, with critics from a wide variety of perspectives arguing that it fails to respect the dignity and separateness of persons, and violates individual rights in pursuance of (varying interpretations of) the 'greater good' (see Kymlicka, 2002; Smart and Williams, 1973; Goodin, 1993). Robert Nozick (1974) and Ronald Dworkin (1977) have criticised utilitarianism in this vein, though with very different ideas about the kinds of inviolable rights people have. Indeed, Rawls' (1971/1999) celebrated theory of 'justice as fairness', and its deployment of the famous 'veil of ignorance' behind which the principles of the just society would be determined by rational actors, was framed explicitly as a critique of utilitarianism. According to Rawls, people would not agree to utilitarian principles which fail 'to take seriously the distinction between persons' (p.163) and endorse 'sacrificial' policies that harm some in order to benefit others. A further significant objection to utilitarianism is that it oversimplifies morality, reducing all human values and objectives to a single scale (Macintyre, 1981/2007), and that it is based on shallow economistic reasoning, tending to elevate material prosperity above all other societal goals, including the fair distribution of income and wealth (see Kymlicka, 2002; Goodin, 1993, and below).

However, utilitarianism is arguably a badly misunderstood moral theory, often caricatured by its opponents (Goodin, 1993) but also sometimes poorly defended and explained by its proponents (Kristjánsson, 2005, 2002). Take, for example, the perception that utilitarian thinking is necessarily closely aligned with 'neoliberal' economic policies that favour a wealthy elite. On the contrary, logically built into utilitarianism is a 'rationale for a more rather than less egalitarian distribution of goods and resources' (p.247), given the 'prioritarianism' implied by declining marginal utility, and the fact that the 'privileged' elite served by such an economic order will by definition be exceedingly small compared to the majority disadvantaged by it (Kymlicka, 2002). Furthermore, utilitarianism is emphatically *only* concerned with material prosperity and wealth insofar as it pays dividends for human welfare, not as an end in itself (Goodin, 1993). For example, utilitarian ideas are currently finding voice via the 'effective altruist' movement, with calls on those wishing 'to make a difference' to 'do good better' (MacAskill, 2015; Singer, 2015). Far from fuelling conspicuous consumption, these ideas have prompted effective altruists to engage in what would usually be considered supererogatory acts, like donating large proportions (e.g. 50%) of their salary on an ongoing basis to demonstrably effective global charities. As Fitzpatrick and Stephens (1999) note, utilitarianism is 'open to some obvious objections ... But few would question that welfare maximisation should form a significant component of public policy' (p.420).

There are a range of potential utilitarian arguments in favour of conduct conditionality, some of which relate to the financial costs to society as a whole (and taxpayers in particular) of, for instance, having large numbers of people receiving welfare benefits (Paz-Fuchs, 2008). There are also utilitarian arguments in favour of intervening to tackle, for example, anti-social behaviour in order to protect the wellbeing of those directly affected by such behaviour (Fitzpatrick and Johnsen, 2009). Furthermore, overall societal welfare may increase if sufficient numbers of citizens derive enough utility from seeing welfare benefits distributed subject to conditions that they view as 'fair' (see below; and Miller, 1992; Goodin, 2002; Taylor Gooby, 2005).

The fundamental point of relevance here is that, as a consequentialist theory, the strength or weakness of the utilitarian case for welfare conditionality turns largely on the empirical questions considered in the last chapter. Can conduct-focused conditions on the receipt of welfare be shown *in fact* to increase the overall sum of human welfare? As demonstrated in Chapter 5, evidence for the positive impacts of welfare conditionality is very often inconsistent, contradictory or lacking. Current data suggests a small number of examples of conditional programmes – some CCTs, immunization-focused conditionality in Australia and intensive 'family intervention projects' tackling anti-social behaviour in the UK – that appear to achieve tangible benefits for those targeted and society at large, but our review of evidence far more frequently backs a utilitarian scepticism regarding the ethicality of conditionality.

Moreover, any potential utility gains associated with conditionality have to be weighed against the negative impacts that such policies may have on those directly targeted – for instance, the stress, material hardship and even destitution that may be experienced by sanctioned jobseekers and their families – and on those whose wellbeing is negatively affected by observing or dealing with these negative impacts (e.g. welfare rights advisers and the 'sympathetic public'). The 'disutility' associated with seeing 'innocent third parties' (Deacon, 2004, p.916) harmed by conditionality in particular must be taken into account, and could be sizable given the moral concern usually reserved for children. Furthermore, declining marginal utility implies that losses to the (typically) low-income groups in receipt of benefits should carry greater moral force than any gains of a similar magnitude to the rest of the population. There are also a range of financial – and sometimes sizable – costs associated with the administration of welfare conditionality that must be weighed in the balance.

All of these points serve to undermine the utilitarian case for conditionality in some areas of welfare policy (and indeed provide significant ammunition for its critics), but depending on the empirical facts the utilitarian rationale *for* conditionality may well be strong in other instances. If the evidence clearly demonstrates substantial utilitarian gains, especially for vulnerable groups, the burden of proof might be argued to be on conditionality's critics to establish why a conditional approach is nevertheless subject to moral opprobrium.

## Contractualism

More common even than utilitarian justifications for conduct conditionality, certainly in the UK, are arguments based on the *contractualist* idea that, in return for welfare assistance, claimants must do all that they can to find work and cease their dependence on benefits. 'Rooted in the concept of reciprocity' (Miscampbell, 2014, p.8), the idea of 'welfare contractualism' has been central to the evolution of more conditional approaches to welfare since the late 1980s (White, 2003; Deacon, 2004; Sage, 2012). It has also been described as 'a fundamental challenge to the dominant intellectual tradition in British social policy and administration, that of the social rights of citizenship formulated by T. H. Marshall' (King, 1999, p.233, see also Dwyer, 2004).

At its core, 'welfare contractualism' imagines the relationship between the citizen and the state as based on a reciprocal agreement involving mutual obligations on both sides so that, if the state is providing 'relief' or assistance, beneficiaries must 'give something back' (Paz-Fuchs, 2008). Or in Deacon's words, 'If the government keeps its part of the bargain, then the claimants should keep theirs' (Deacon, 2004, p.915). It also links to a particular conceptualisation of social justice or 'fairness' (that extends far beyond the political Right, and indeed into Marxist thought) which alights on desert as a principal moral criterion for the allocation of societal goods, with deservingness defined as 'responsible behaviour', and often more narrowly as preparedness to make a societal contribution via paid work (White, 2003; Miller, 1999; and see below).

As well as this emphasis on citizens' responsibility to contribute to society through paid work, fainter echoes of contractualism are present in other welfare spheres; for example, the requirement that potentially homeless people ought to do all that they can to resolve their own housing problems under the 'Housing Options' models of homelessness prevention that are now applied across the UK, and in the 'Acceptable Behaviour Agreements' and other instruments used in some anti-social behaviour programmes to define the responsibilities of perpetrators (see Chapter 4).

This 'something for something' model of contractualism has an intuitive moral appeal, with reciprocity 'ubiquitous in anthropological accounts of morality' (Graham et al., 2011, p.368), and central to the whole concept of 'social insurance' benefits. Contractualism understood in these terms can moreover claim an association with the highly influential theory of 'justice as fairness' developed by John Rawls (1971/1999), within the tradition of Kant and Rousseau. In developing his theory, Rawls emphasises the importance of both reciprocity and mutual benefit. He recognises, however, that any such emphasis begs the question of whether the state, and indeed society more generally, is in fact 'keeping its side of the bargain', explaining that 'one has a duty to uphold just arrangements, and an obligation to do one's part when one has accepted a position in them' (Rawls, 1971/1999, p.275). On this view, any such obligation to 'do one's part' weakens, or breaks down entirely, when 'unjust arrangements' prevail. Gough (1998) has argued in a similar vein that 'It is contradictory to ask of someone that they fulfil their social duties, yet to deny them the prerequisite need satisfaction which will enable them to do so' (p.52).

Building on Rawlsian foundations, Stuart White's (2003) *The Civic Minimum* develops an explicitly egalitarian conceptualisation of welfare contractualism which focuses on 'conditions of fair reciprocity'. For White, this includes the elimination of 'brute luck' poverty, the reduction of inequalities of opportunity, and protection against discrimination. While he holds that citizens have 'potentially enforceable obligations to make a productive contribution to the community', these obligations arise only in a society honouring an 'income adequacy' criterion, wherein citizens engaged in a minimum standard of productive participation earn 'a sufficiently generous share of the social product' (White, 2003, p.17).

The force of the contractualist case for welfare conditionality thus appears to depend on the realities of social arrangements in a particular context, and it is far from clear that the necessary arrangements pertain in many of the places in both the Global North and South considered in this book where welfare conditionality currently operates. In the UK case specifically, one could certainly question whether the required civic minimum currently exists. In part this relates to the very low (and eroding) value of working-age benefits (Hood and Waters, 2017b) and to the growth in 'in-work poverty' and 'exclusionary employment' (Bailey, 2018), both of which pose challenges for White's income adequacy criterion.

Declining social mobility in recent years (Social Mobility Commission, 2016), together with profoundly unequal risks of experiencing poverty (Bramley and Bailey, 2018) and strongly associated forms of exclusion such as homelessness (Bramley and Fitzpatrick, 2017), also speak to an inequality of opportunity that plays a very large part in shaping *who* is poor, and therefore likely to find themselves subject to various forms of welfare conditionality (see also Pérez-Muñoz, 2017). With the odds stacked much more heavily against some people than others, and 'irrefutable evidence that an individual's life chances are seriously diminished by the experience of childhood poverty and deprivation' (Deacon, 2004, p.920), it is difficult to argue that the 'background conditions' for fair reciprocity pertain (White, 2003). Indeed, writing after the ramping up of conditionality since *The Civic Minimum* was published, White (2017) has shifted to a highly sceptical orientation regarding its ethical legitimacy, offering support instead to the growing interest in many countries in an 'unconditional basic income'. He explains:

> since background conditions for fair reciprocity are not satisfied, and there is a serious risk that they will not be satisfied in the future, we should proceed on the assumption that conditionality is likely to be unjust for the foreseeable future and, given the dangers from unjust conditionality, seek to move away from it as much as we can.
>
> *(p.191)*

As noted above, such arguments against conditionality are bolstered by the evident asymmetry between the conditions attached to public welfare focused on the middle classes as compared to that imposed on low-income households in many advanced welfare contexts.

## Communitarianism

Communitarians, or in Deacon's terms 'mutualists', share with contractualists an emphasis on people's obligations to contribute to society. However, they reject the liberal individualism that underpins welfare contractualism, and what they view as its overemphasis on personal freedoms at the expense of community solidarity and social cohesion (see Mulhall and Swift, 1996; Etzioni, 1998; Kymlicka, 2002). For communitarians, people have responsibilities towards each other that arise *independently* of any claims that they can make on government. These obligations are therefore rooted not in any 'bargain' between individuals and the state, but rather in principles of mutual respect and recognition of the needs of others, and our pre-existing 'personal responsibility for the common good' (Selznick, 1998, p.63).

There are a number of diverse, even opposing, strands of communitarianism. Thus, 'backward looking communitarianism', associated with nostalgia for traditional values and a loss of a sense of community, appeals to traditional Conservatives and anti-egalitarians (Phillips, 1993). A far-Left version, on the other hand, is encapsulated in the Marxist vision of the post-capitalist society (Dwyer, 2010). Other strands of mutualism are associated with Christian or theological principles that stress human interdependence and obligations to care for the 'needy other' (Johnsen et al., forthcoming). What all communitarians have in common is a distrust of personal liberty as a good in itself, and an inclination to elevate their (often contradictory) visions of the collective good over individual freedom or wellbeing.

It is clearly well within the scope of this normative perspective – indeed it is desirable – that the state take on an 'active' and 'interventionist' role in promoting (through sanctions, incentives or other social control mechanisms) ways of life that are deemed to be in line with communal shared values (Mulhall and Swift, 1996). Communitarianism can therefore readily be brought to bear as a normative framework within which conditional approaches to welfare are justified as a means of enforcing community norms with regard, for example, to undertaking paid work, refraining from anti-social behaviour, ensuring that one's children attend school, accepting relevant healthcare interventions, and so on.

Moreover, as White (2003) explains, from the communitarian viewpoint, the obligations citizens owe each other arise merely from their membership of a community, notwithstanding the fact that they may have had little choice about joining that community, and are not contingent on state intervention to lessen material inequalities or achieve any specific 'civic minimum' (see also Deacon, 2004). Though modern communitarians are not *necessarily* as antagonistic towards equality as they are towards individual liberty, their distributive goals tend to be limited to minimising 'social exclusion' in the interests of maintaining an acceptable level of 'social cohesion', with some theorists in this vein even emphasising that 'inequality as such is not the issue' (Selznick, 1998, quoted in Deacon, 2004, p.918). John Gray (2000), for example, argues that 'social inclusion' requires that every member of a society has access to its central goods, and that this requirement incorporates two components – fair opportunities and the satisfaction of basic needs. Once these requirements are met, distribution is irrelevant. In his view, while there may be large areas of practical agreement between egalitarians and 'inclusionists', they subscribe to distinct ideals which, although sometimes overlapping, can also be competitors:

> Supporters of social inclusion do not pursue an ideal of egalitarian justice, but an ideal of common life. This will surely condemn many inequalities. But not all.
>
> *(Gray, 2000, p.22)*

It can be seen, therefore, that communitarian or mutualist justifications for welfare conditionality are likely to be found persuasive only by those who place relatively little store by matters of personal liberty and/or equality. As Deacon (2004) comments:

> The most serious limitation of the mutualist argument ... is its failure to recognise that the responsibilities of the affluent go beyond the provision of ... a 'baseline equality of condition' ... the conception of the good society that underpins mutualism itself ... requires a more equal distribution of material resources than is presently the case in Britain – or indeed in the USA.
>
> *(p.920)*

But for the communitarian, this is to put the cart before the horse. If dominant social values see distribution according to conduct as ethically desirable, and inequality as ethically unproblematic, these empirical facts are sufficient *in and of themselves* to justify conditionality, even in the most extremely unequal of contexts. Such a perspective begs the question, of course, of where dominant social values come from (they may be driven by privileged elites, for instance; see O'Grady, 2017). Communitarianism nevertheless offers, for those who find its logic appealing, an exceedingly clear justification of welfare conditionality, likely the strongest of all of the normative perspectives considered in this chapter.

## Paternalism

Some justifications of welfare conditionality take a quite different tack, arguing that these measures are in the best interests of the welfare claimants themselves, with such 'paternalistic' justifications said to be motivated by 'a beneficent concern for [the] welfare [of those targeted]' (Scoccia, 2008, p.352). Paternalists share with communitarians the emphasis on an activist state, but with less focus on the enforcement of obligations owed to the community as a whole, and more on ensuring compliance with behavioural patterns in order to protect people from the consequences of their own poor decision making. 'Hard paternalism' uses forceful or coercive methods, such as benefit sanctions, to induce people to act in ways that are argued to be in their own interests, whereas libertarian paternalism seeks to non-coercively 'nudge' people towards such behaviours (Thaler and Sunstein, 2008, and see Chapter 5), and can be understood as a form of 'soft paternalism' alongside influence and (rational) persuasion (Grant, 2012).

The best-known advocate of hard paternalism linked to work obligations is the American conservative Lawrence Mead, whose ideas were discussed in detail in Chapter 4. According to Mead (1992), long-term welfare recipients are not competent self-regarding individuals who will act rationally, but rather dependents who ought to receive support on condition of certain restrictions imposed by a 'tutelary' state (see also Deacon, 2004). Mead believes that the behavioural responses of low-income welfare recipients are shaped not so much by economic incentives as by the exercise of stern 'authority' that uncompromisingly signals the community's normative expectations that they do all they can to move off welfare and into work (or at least off welfare).

Trading off short-term pain for future gain is more broadly a key feature of paternalist justifications for interventions which seek to 'save people from themselves'. Even quite severe benefit sanctions that are acknowledged to cause short-term hardship to welfare recipients, and to innocent third parties in their households, especially their children (Deacon, 2004), are argued from this perspective to be in the long-term best interests of these low-income families, as it encourages them to free themselves from poverty and welfare dependency. Dunn (2014), for instance, lists amongst his reasons for having 'fewer qualms than some commentators about imposing severe benefit sanctions on people who do not comply with welfare conditions' (p.194) that it 'develops people's work habits and skills', thus increasing their future employment chances, and thereby promises 'to increase the incomes of the poorest households, in order to help improve their lives' (p.194) (see, however, ample evidence on the growing prevalence of in-work poverty in the UK: Bailey, 2018; Tinson et al., 2016). In the recent literature, Perkins (2016) has perhaps gone furthest in providing the groundwork for this paternalist justification, in making the highly controversial argument that long-term benefit receipt, or growing up in a 'welfare dependent' household, is associated with developing an 'Employment-Resistant Personality Profile', characterised by an 'aggressive, antisocial and rule-breaking predisposition' (p.3; see also Lambert, 2016; Foster, 2016).

However, possibly in part because of its associations with Right-wing theorists such as Mead, Dunn and Perkins, and also because of the suspicion that those who offer these sorts of justifications for conditional forms of welfare are often in reality hypocritically serving their own class interests (Fletcher and Wright, 2017; Lambert, 2016), the pejorative connotation of paternalism in social policy debate is now so overwhelming that it can seem almost impossible to mount a reasoned defence of it (Parsell and Marston, 2016).

Paternalistic interventions arouse such ire because they infringe the key liberal principle that people are best placed to know their own interests (New, 1999). But Gregory (2015) and Parsell and Marston (2016) have recently and persuasively argued that there is a case for some rehabilitation of the concept of 'justifiable paternalism' in the case of certain vulnerable groups who are not well placed to make autonomous decisions regarding their own welfare, at least in the short term. Rough sleepers suffering from life-limiting, and often life-threatening, severe addiction and/or mental ill health are an obvious case in point, where their ability to exercise meaningful autonomy is severely compromised by the debilitating effects of these conditions on their cognitive capacity to make decisions and/or look towards the future (Epel et al., 1999; Sullivan et al., 2010). The key (empirical) question raised is whether paternalistic restriction in short-term freedom of action can be demonstrated to restore, or establish, at least a basic level of personal autonomy for extremely vulnerable adults in circumstances where this would otherwise be absent or threatened (Watts et al., 2017; Caplan, 2008). As discussed in Chapter 4, there is some evidence that is supportive of this position in the case of street homeless people, though it is mixed and somewhat inconclusive.

With regard to paternalistic justifications for welfare conditionality more broadly, too, there is a fundamental empirical question about the data available to establish that the short-term hardship associated with benefit sanctions, for example, is *in fact* outweighed by longer-term gains for welfare recipients in terms of labour market participation, rewards and general wellbeing. As discussed in Chapter 5, the data available to support this proposition is far from compelling, though a more persuasive case may be made for certain kinds of CCTs in the developing world. We would argue, therefore, that even leaving aside the in-principle objections to paternalism that liberals may have, the most basic evidential requirements for justifying welfare conditionality from this perspective (other than perhaps with respect to exceptionally vulnerable adults) remains unsatisfied.

## Social justice

The idea of social justice pertains to fundamental questions regarding the distribution of society's benefits and burdens – 'who should get what and why?' Theories of social justice employ a range of criteria in promoting a moral basis for the distribution of society's valued goods, including merit, desert and need (Johnston, 2011; Miller, 1999). However, most are egalitarian in some fundamental sense (Sen, 1992), concerned with minimising inequalities in some relevant 'space', such as access to 'primary goods' (Rawls, 1971/1999), 'capabilities' (Sen, 1992) or 'resources' (Dworkin, 2000). Increasing theoretical and policy attention is also now paid to equality of 'recognition' and 'respect' for different social groups (Young, 1990). While many social justice theorists lay emphasis on certain kinds of 'basic rights' (Rawls, 1971/1999; Miller, 1999), this normative lens generally lends itself to a strongly consequentialist (though not utilitarian) orientation, given its focus on the achievement of relevant *distributive outcomes*, though some social justice analysts concede that *procedural justice* has an independent value of its own (Miller, 1999).

One modern account of social justice which captures a compelling combination of many of the qualities noted above is that of David Miller (1999). Miller starts from the deeply democratic premise that any worthwhile ethical system has to be at least *plausible* to the general public, which is not the same thing as saying (as communitarians risk) that theories of justice should simply mirror their prejudices: 'A theory of justice has to do more than simply report popular beliefs . . . it must also show that the principles in question are philosophically coherent and can be welded together to form a cohesive whole' (p.245). This is in keeping with the Rawlsian ethical method which seeks to achieve 'reflective equilibrium' between normative theory and pre-theoretical moral intuitions. As Miller explains, his aim is to

> discover the underlying principles that people use when they judge some aspect of their society to be just or unjust, and then to show that these principles are coherent, both separately and when taken together ... If we want to describe what social justice means in contemporary political debate, then sooner rather than later we must look at what the people themselves think.
>
> *(p.ix)*

A method for meeting the strong empirical requirements of such an approach is already provided by moral psychologists' development of Moral Foundations Theory discussed above (see also Graham et al., 2011). But the task of Rawls and Miller as philosophers extends considerably beyond this 'purely descriptive perspective' (Graham et al., 2011, p.380), asking how can we reconcile the varying and sometimes contradictory principles (Harm/Care, Fairness/Reciprocity, Ingroup/Loyalty, Authority/Respect, and Purity/Sanctity) implicated in popular conceptions of social justice?

Miller's solution is to exploit the fact that people draw on different principles from their 'moral repertoire' in considering the ethicality of distributions of *particular goods* in *distinct circumstances*. Thus, according to Miller, social justice requires, first, that each person's *needs* be met according to a common standard recognised across the relevant society. This is not simply a matter of ensuring that everyone reaches as a socially-defined minimum, but rather that 'need-meeting resources must be distributed according to need, in other words, there should be no preventable inequalities in the extent to which different people's needs are met' (Miller, 1999, p.258). Following Amartya Sen (1992), he argues that such need-meeting resources are best defined as a set of 'functionings' that 'together make up a minimally decent life for people in the society in question' (p.247; for an alternative conception of basic needs, see Doyal and Gough, 1991). Miller's model echoes in broad terms, though it is somewhat more strongly egalitarian in orientation, the 'consensual' approach to the definition of poverty and deprivation that is now dominant in social science in the UK (Bramley and Bailey, 2018).

However, second, and controversially for many on the political Left, Miller also argues that 'Justice requires that many social resources be allocated to individuals on the basis of *desert*' (1999, p.248; emphasis added). The main issue here is 'economic desert' – how people are rewarded for the work they perform. He lays emphasis on the importance of equal opportunities in the labour market and on regulatory regimes that promote meritocratic outcomes as far as possible, acting to 'dampen rather than to amplify the effects of luck' (p.249). While he also acknowledges that the current magnitude of inequality in incomes (and we might add wealth) in most capitalist societies is too great to be compatible with the requirements of justice, and that needs must always be met, he insists that beyond this a 'just distribution of income would be substantially unequal' (p.249).

Finally, Miller takes the position that, in their capacity as citizens, people must be treated as *equals*, and that this requires that they enjoy equal access to a range of legal, political and social rights (hinting at a deontological strand in his thinking), but also that public policy should give equal consideration to the interests of all those affected by it (implying a more utilitarian perspective). While he is sympathetic to the institutionalisation of social rights via formal constitutional requirements, Miller suggests caution in not overstating the capacity of constitutional mechanisms, conceding that 'it may be hard to specify the content of the[se] right[s] in such a way that a judicial body can determine whether a particularly policy fulfils the right or not' (p.250; see also Fitzpatrick et al., 2014). He therefore urges democratic as well as legal decision-making processes that support equal consideration of interests and preferences, especially for minority groups.

Miller's theory is only one interpretation of the complex concept of social justice. However, it is an attractive and pragmatic model, recognising as it does that norms of reciprocity, desert and merit exert a powerful ethical pull, alongside principles of equality and need, and drawing them together into an integrated and defensible whole which is context-sensitive and democratically grounded.

Leading social justice theorists – including Rawls (1971/1999) as well as Miller (1999) – make the point that their theories of distributional justice are most relevant in conditions of 'relative' or 'moderate' scarcity. In conditions of absolute scarcity – where citizens' basic needs cannot feasibly be met by any distribution of the total available resources – a determined emphasis on utility maximisation via economic growth may be more appropriate than a thoroughgoing emphasis on the detailed distribution of resources. However, in the context of the already-rich societies of the Western world, our long-term 'love affair' with economic growth, so often prioritised over distributive questions of equality and justice, not to mention environmental sustainability, is on the face of it more difficult to justify (Wilkinson, 2005).

For this reason, and because conceptualisations of social justice like Miller's incorporate many of the most compelling elements of the other normative perspectives considered above, one could argue that this is an especially relevant normative lens through which to assess the ethical defensibility of welfare conditionality in wealthy countries like the UK. So are key examples of conduct conditionality considered in this book socially just when tested against Miller's principles? Even a cursory analysis of the available empirical data is sufficient to indicate that very often they are not, because they involve the 'desert' criterion being applied to goods that should, according to his theory, be 'desert-insensitive' and allocated purely on the basis of need.

The core needs highlighted by Miller as required for minimally adequate 'functionings' include access to adequate food and shelter, reflecting one obvious interpretation of the importance of 'harm' in the moral concerns of populations across the globe (Graham et al., 2011), and reflecting too the view of the general UK public in a recent study of 'destitution' in the UK (Fitzpatrick et al., 2016). This same study found that, in part as a result of welfare conditionality – and specifically benefit sanctions – significant numbers of UK citizens were rendered completely destitute, and that going without food was the most commonly experienced deprivation experienced by these households. This clearly breaches Miller's principles of justice, as conditionality in this case is leading to basic nutritional needs being left unmet. Links between sanctioning and food insecurity have frequently been made in the broader evidence base on conditionality in the UK and US (see Chapter 5), with media reports in the UK suggesting an association with the untimely deaths of some of those recently deemed 'fit for work' under the intensified conditionality regime now in place for sick and disabled people (Ryan, 2015).

It should be noted, however, returning to the debates in Chapter 2, that this deleterious (and perhaps in some cases tragic) impact of behavioural conditionality should be viewed in the wider context of other key characteristics of welfare systems, and in particular their generosity. In the UK, it has been shown that the level of income maintenance benefits paid to unemployed under-25-year-olds living away from the family home is insufficient to raise income above a publically-endorsed destitution level (Fitzpatrick et al., 2016), and thus their injustice in Miller's terms arises not only from their conditional nature, but also because the base amount of the relevant cash transfer is insufficient to allow fundamental needs to be met. Where such base rates are higher and/or the proportion of benefit income sanctioned lower, these extreme impacts would be far less likely to occur.

As housing, or at least shelter, of an adequate standard may also be considered a basic need in Miller's framework, this normative perspective also condemns as unjust some conditional aspects of UK housing and homelessness policies. This includes both some non-behavioural forms of conditionality (e.g. the exclusion of single homeless people from entitlement to even temporary accommodation when faced with the prospect of sleeping rough; see Fitzpatrick and Pawson, 2016) and some behavioural aspects (e.g. the application of 'intentionality' criteria to exclude some homeless households to access to long-term rehousing on the basis of 'feckless' conduct). This housing-focused critique also extends to benefit conditionality, which has now been shown to both cause homelessness (including in its most severe manifestations) and frustrate its resolution (Batty et al., 2015).

The pluralist social justice framework offered here establishes a fairly high bar for welfare conditionality to pass in order to be ethically justified. But, unlike the rights-based perspectives considered at the beginning of this chapter, it does not offer an unqualified critique of conditionality. The high priority given to meeting needs/safeguarding 'functionings', for instance, is at least consistent with – and might in fact ethically mandate – forms of conditionality that demonstrably 'safeguard the future autonomy of people ... facing life-threatening challenges'

(Watts et al., 2017, p.13). It thus allows for some of the most compelling insights offered by paternalist and utilitarian perspectives, without requiring buy-in to the more controversial aspects of their underlying logic.

## Concluding comments

This chapter has argued for a pluralistic approach to normative social policy analysis rather than a monist emphasis on rights, utility maximisation or any single ethical perspective. This is rooted in an acknowledgment that the 'good society' has to be judged according to multiple criteria rather than a single standard, with a balance having to be struck between a range of (often competing) societal objectives such as the protection of personal liberty, the advancement of social justice, the nurturing of social cohesion, the pursuit of economic prosperity and the establishment and institutionalisation of democracy.

It is important to resist the reductionist tendency apparent in some strands of philosophical endeavour, not least because the worst sorts of societies tend to give absolute priority (at least in theory) to just one of these objectives above all others (King, 2011). Monist approaches can also be obfuscatory in their intellectual impact. As Miller (1999) argues:

> the centrality of social justice to contemporary political debate should not induce us to pack into this concept everything we might find socially desirable ... to assimilate distinct political ideals to one another is not only to court confusion, but to obscure the need for choices that involve some sacrifice of one value, which might be justice itself, in the name of others – democracy, individuality, or social harmony.
>
> *(p.17)*

It is thus in the spirit of Isaiah Berlin's (1969) and Michael Ignatieff's (2000) 'value pluralism' that we argue for a multi-faceted normative perspective on welfare conditionality that lays emphasis on the interdependence between ethical reasoning and empirical evidence in settling moral questions in this field. Such an approach can help to counter the tendency for some social policy analysts to bypass the issue of trade-offs by focusing on only one value (fairness, rights), and for

some economists to do likewise (utility maximisation, material prosperity). The moral pluralist position of Berlin holds that such trade-offs are not simply an outcome of scarcity and competition for resources. Rather, even in a context of abundance, 'tragic' policy choices are required between legitimate but incommensurable goals because values themselves can conflict, e.g. generous social welfare payments versus work incentives, or targeting need versus reducing stigma.

How persuasive or 'legitimate' one finds each of the specific normative perspectives discussed in this chapter will depend largely on one's own personal political outlook and values, and underpinning 'moral concerns'. Most people will be attracted to more than one of them, to at least some extent, and weigh some combination of them in the balance in assessing the moral case for specific forms and instances of conditionality. For example, paternalist justifications for state intervention in the form of incentives and sanctions may weigh more heavily with vulnerable groups, such as homeless people with mental health problems, whereas norms of reciprocity may be to the fore where it is felt that people are well equipped to 'pay their dues', but are electing instead to free ride.

Notwithstanding this pluralist perspective, it is important to note that the normative lenses discussed in this chapter interrelate in at least two important senses. First, at a conceptual level they are often cross-referring frameworks – e.g. respect for certain types of rights can sometimes be justified by reference to the fact that this leads to good utilitarian outcomes. Second, empirically they can point to the same substantive conclusions, but for different, or only partially coterminous, reasons.

In fact, it is very often the case that welfare interventions can be justified, or opposed, from a range of normative perspectives simultaneously, and such 'moral triangulation' can be argued to significantly increase the persuasiveness of the case for, or against, particular forms of conditionality. Deacon (2004), for example, concluded that a 'powerful case' (p.912) for justifying Labour's anti-social behaviour policies could be mounted via a combination of contractualism, paternalism and, especially, mutualism, even though any one of these justifications on their own would have been insufficient in his view. On the other hand, as should be evident from the discussion above, there are weighty objections to benefit sanctions, particularly in their more

severe manifestations, that may be mounted from contractualist, utilitarian, paternalist and social justice perspectives, as well as by employing 'rights-talk'. This triangulated form of ethical interrogation can provide significant ballast for specific substantive conclusions reached on particular aspects of welfare conditionality, and also conveys a democratic respect for the multiple, divergent and contextualised ethical impulses evident across society.

In the next and final chapter of the book, we will attempt to draw the threads of the normative analysis offered in this chapter, together with the empirical evidence discussed in earlier chapters, to suggest an integrated approach to assessing the *efficacy* and *ethicality* of conditional approaches to welfare provision and practice.

## Note

1 The terms 'moral' and 'ethical' are often used interchangeably, but 'moral' can also be understood to have narrower meaning, which pertains to norms about how one ought to treat other people (morals are therefore 'other-regarding'); 'ethical' can be understood more broadly as encompassing 'living a life well lived', including themes of self-improvement, cultural enrichment and other 'self-regarding' issues in addition to other-regarding concerns.

# 7
# CONCLUSIONS

This book set out to 'map' the contemporary terrain associated with welfare conditionality, addressing the myriad conceptual, empirical and normative questions that it poses. While the intensification of conditionality in Western welfare systems, and in the UK in particular, is the main focus of the book, we have also made relevant connections with the rolling out of conditional forms of welfare across the Global South.

The early chapters sought to set conditionality in its appropriate context – as one way in which welfare states and specific policies diverge – and to 'deconstruct' behavioural conditionality into its constituent parts, describing the manifold ways in which its design, objectives, implementation and stringency vary. We also offered a detailed exploration of the application of conditionality to four key target groups – unemployed people (including young people and sick and disabled people), low-income families with children, social housing tenants and homeless people – highlighting the diversity of underpinning rationales and conditional mechanisms employed. In so doing, we hope to have helped broaden debates on conditionality, which are often highly polarised, even inflammatory, in tone and content.

Throughout the book our main focus has been on those aspects of the welfare system and conditionality that are most likely to affect poor or otherwise marginalised populations. It is within this territory that the ethical and policy dilemmas associated with conditionality are most troubling and contentious. The book is ultimately concerned with the *efficacy* and *ethical legitimacy* of welfare conditionality as applied to these groups, two matters that, though conceptually distinct, are in practice inextricably linked.

The remainder of this concluding chapter will consider our overarching findings on these two key points, before drawing the threads together from across the entire book to propose a framework for systematic evaluation of conditional welfare approaches. We finish the chapter, and the book, with a reminder of the broader context within which all considerations of welfare conditionality must sit.

## Putting conditionality in the spotlight

Our overriding conclusion with regard to the matter of *efficacy* is that there is not, nor can there be, a single answer to the question 'does welfare conditionality "work"?' The sheer diversity of techniques, subjects and impacts of conditionality examined in this book give the lie to any notion that there could be a simple 'yes or no' answer to such a question.

Furthermore, and crucially, consideration of whether any specific policy intervention 'works' turns fundamentally on the 'end' which is sought. If one's objective is simply to 'hassle' people out of the benefit system, then sanction-backed conditionality certainly can be shown to work (Mead, 2005). If, on the other hand, one's ultimate aim is to increase the chances that unemployed people will make an early and sustainable re-entry to the labour market, and in so doing enhance the quality of life for them and their families, then the evidence for benefit conditionality and sanctions is, at best, extremely mixed.

Such behaviourally-focused agendas also, of course, rely on the prior (and highly contentious) assumption that unemployed people's conduct and mind-set is the fundamental problem that needs to be 'fixed' in order to increase employment rates. As Bramley and Bailey (2018) comment:

> If you believe that whether people are working or not is more a matter of choice than opportunity, and that there are not

> structural barriers of geography and discrimination which make it much more difficult for some people to find work, then you are more likely to favour welfare policies which impose conditions and create incentives for working-age people to actively seek work.
>
> *(p.352)*

However, many analysts dispute this sort of stance, arguing that such 'supply side' measures miss the point completely, misdiagnosing 'structural' problems of economic and industrial decline as attributable to psychological or behavioural 'deficits' on the part of unemployed people (Friedli and Stearn, 2015; Watson, 2015; Beatty and Fothergill, 2013, 2016a, 2016b; Bramley et al., 2015).

At the same time, and alongside the ideological controversies and inconclusive evidence base surrounding out-of-work benefit conditionality in developed welfare states, there are other examples, particularly from the Global South, of conditional welfare interventions that have been demonstrably effective in meeting their programme objectives to reduce poverty and/or promote engagement with education or health provision (Bastagli, 2009; Fiszbein et al., 2009). Even here, though, what is not always clear is whether the conditionality of such programmes is core to achieving these positive outcomes (Pellerano and Barca, 2014; Kidd, 2016), or whether non-conditional approaches (unconditional income transfers, the provision of information, improved access to education, enhanced support) would be equally as effective (Dhaliwal et al., 2014; Singer, 2015). A quite different sort of example is provided by 'interventionist' policies focused on vulnerable people involved in life-limiting (or life-threatening) behaviour, such as chronic rough sleeping and/or serious drug misuse, that have shown positive results in some cases (Johnsen and Fitzpatrick, 2010). But responses to these interventions can be unpredictable, potentially driving vulnerable people further away from support, and have thus been characterised as 'high risk' (Johnsen and Fitzpatrick, 2007).

We have also argued that it is unlikely, even implausible, that a 'universal' conclusion about the *ethical legitimacy* (or not) of conditional forms of welfare provision can be reached. This arises in part from the meta-ethical perspective that we have adopted in this book, which might broadly be characterised as 'value pluralism' in the tradition of Isaiah Berlin (1969). This stance recognises that the 'good society' should be judged according to multiple criteria rather than a single standard, with a balance having to be struck between a range of legitimate (yet often competing) societal objectives. These 'high-level' societal objectives may include, for example, the protection of personal liberty, the advancement of social justice, the nurturing of social cohesion, the pursuit of economic prosperity, and the establishment and institutionalisation of democracy and/or citizen 'empowerment' (Fitzpatrick et al., 2002; Kintrea, 2006).

In this spirit, we explored the defensibility of welfare conditionality from a range of established normative perspectives, including rights-based theories, utilitarianism, contractualism, communitarianism, paternalism and social justice. We argued that how persuasive one finds each of these perspectives will depend largely on one's own personal political outlook and underpinning 'moral foundations' (Haidt and Graham, 2007), with most people attracted to more than one of them, to at least some extent, and weighing a combination of them in the balance in assessing the moral case for specific forms and instances of conditionality.

However, a key point to emphasise here is that, whichever one or combination of these normative frameworks one gives precedence to, there is an interdependence between ethical reasoning and empirical evidence in settling moral questions pertaining to the justifiability or otherwise of conditionality. In some cases, this interdependence is extremely strong. For example, a utilitarian will want to know whether, in reality, conditional measures do indeed maximise utility (however defined), while a rights theorist will be concerned to examine how conditional forms of welfare in practice violate the rights they hold to be fundamental. A contractualist – if they are of an egalitarian bent – will want to explore whether the background conditions of 'fair reciprocity' have in fact been met. Likewise, a paternalist will seek to establish if the policies in question in reality serve the best interests of those targeted by them, while someone with a social justice orientation will want to pay close attention to the distributive outcomes of specific conditional welfare approaches. Even communitarians, whose focus on upholding community norms stretches furthest towards favouring conditionality regardless of its consequences, may have an empirical job on their hands to establish what those norms actually are, and be driven to a consideration of impacts where no clear normative consensus exists. It follows, then, that for the most part we cannot fully assess the ethical defensibility of any particular conditional intervention without empirical research taking cognisance of its impacts, both intended and unintended, positive and negative. These impacts vary a great deal in practice, and consequently one's views on the ethical legitimacy of the measures in question may vary as well.

The implication of these core conclusions on matters of both effectiveness and ethical legitimacy is that each particular example of welfare conditionality must be assessed on its own merits, taking full account of the empirical facts, and from the perspective of the relevant range of moral standpoints. What is required, we would suggest, is an assessment framework that is *context-specific* (i.e. is clear about the kind of society, welfare goods and target groups under consideration), *evidence-informed* (i.e. employs robust data on impacts, both intended and unintended) and *ethically-literate* (i.e. makes use of the normative tools and frameworks best suited to systematically exploring the moral implications of conditionality). What such an assessment framework might look like, and how it could be applied, are matters to which we now turn.

## Putting conditionality to the test

Drawing across all of the key themes in the book, we would argue that systematic and ordered attention to the following series of questions can usefully structure an assessment of the efficacy and ethical legitimacy of specific instances of welfare conditionality. While the diverse normative perspectives highlighted above may vary in the intensity with which they lay emphasis on each of these questions, we would argue that virtually all of the questions considered below remain relevant across the range of personal 'moral foundations' (Haidt and Graham, 2007) anchoring any one person's viewpoint.

The first question to be considered, reflecting the fact that this entire conversation is infused with an ethical dimension, is whether the purpose of the behavioural conditionality at issue can be considered *legitimate*

(Grant, 2006, 2012; Watts et al., 2017). 'Effectiveness' in achieving particular ends has no ethical worth in and of itself – it is only of value insofar as the ends being pursued are defensible. It would seem difficult to consider measures pursued with purely punitive intent – as some have claimed to be the case with benefit sanctions (Webster, 2015a; Adler, 2016) and 'revanchist' measures against rough sleepers in US cities (Amster, 2003) – to be legitimate from any plausible ethical orientation. Extreme interpretations of 'communitarianism' claiming strong and straightforward populist desire for such measures might be argued to justify such patently retributive policies, but it is far from clear that public attitudes are so simplistic and consensual (and where they do exist they are highly likely to rest on misunderstandings of the causes and nature of unemployment or homelessness).

Nevertheless, the divergent normative perspectives reviewed in this book would allow for quite a wide range of ends to be considered legitimate from at least one moral angle. What is most interesting, and discriminating, we would suggest is to consider two points: first, can the purpose of the conditional welfare intervention be considered legitimate from *multiple* (rather than just a single) normative perspectives, with distinct moral theories thus triangulating to offer robust and multi-layered justification (see also Deacon, 2004; Gabriel, 2017)? Second, where there is a clash between incommensurate moral values, is pre-eminence being given to the most compelling or appropriate one in that *context*?

On this latter point, we return to Miller's (1999) democratically-grounded approach, with which we have already expressed our sympathy in Chapter 6. Miller's social justice theory foregrounds the fact that people draw on different principles from their 'moral repertoire' in considering the ethicality of distributions of *particular goods* in *distinct circumstances*. Likewise, we would contend that, without seeking to dictate what people's ultimate values ought to be, there are some plausible context-dependent principles that can be applied in determining the applicability of specific normative perspectives and moral criteria focused on, for example:

- *the economic context* – in contexts of *relative* scarcity, such as pertain for the most part in rich Western countries, we would argue that there are compelling moral grounds for giving priority to distributive justice (see Rawls, 1971/1999). In conditions of absolute scarcity the case for a different ordering of priorities (e.g. the prioritisation of utility maximisation via economic growth) may be stronger;

- *the social context* – before one can defensibly invoke contractualist principles in justifying welfare conditionality, we would suggest the need for confirmation that 'background conditions of fair reciprocity' apply in the social and welfare arrangements of the given society (see White, 2003);
- *the goods in question* – following Miller (1999), we would argue that some goods (i.e. those that fulfil basic needs requirements) should be entirely 'desert-insensitive' in their distribution, whereas it may be legitimate for other goods to be distributed according to some measures of individual desert or merit, so long as relevant background conditions are met with regard to equal opportunities and the overall scale of societal inequality. This approach leaves space for particular countries to democratically operationalise 'what counts' as basic need fulfilment above some plausible minimum (Nussbaum, 2000; Bramley and Bailey, 2018);
- *the people/behaviours in question* – we would argue that paternalistic policy objectives should not necessarily be dismissed out of hand, but can be legitimate, and overcome liberal objections, where they can be shown to be autonomy-protecting or enhancing for vulnerable groups (Gregory, 2015; Parsell and Marston, 2016; Watts et al., 2017). Given well-rehearsed and legitimate concerns about paternalist interventions, any such justifications would need to be treated with great care, with a strong emphasis placed on demonstrable benefit to the group in question (see below).

Conditional measures that fail to meet this 'legitimacy of purpose' test, or do so only weakly (i.e. from only one normative perspective, and not necessarily the most compelling one in the given context), cannot be considered ethically justified, though it remains possible for them to be efficacious (in the sense of effectively meeting the illegitimate or semi-legitimate ends they seek).

Second, having established the legitimacy of the ultimate 'end' that a particular measure seeks to achieve, the next task is to examine the *alignment* between the behaviour change sought and the underlying social ill that measure seeks to address. There are cases discussed in this book where the necessary alignment between the ultimate end sought and the behaviour change pursued is clearly present. Examples here include attempts to change the damaging lifestyle of vulnerable rough sleepers in order to protect their health and well-being, and CCTs directly linked to child immunisation programmes. However, as noted above, many would argue that, in at least some labour market contexts, conditionality and sanctions associated with out-of-work benefits fall at this early evaluative hurdle, not least by mistaking a structural problem (weak labour demand) for a behavioural problem (unwillingness to work) (Beatty and Fothergill, 2016a). Any conditionality measure that does not fit this alignment test can be considered neither efficacious nor ethical.

Third is the question of how convincing or otherwise the relevant '*theory of change*' is with regard to the shift in conduct being pursued. In other words, before embarking on any conditional approach, does it seem likely that the policy measures being undertaken – including any threatened sanctions – will bring about the sought-after behaviour change in an acceptably high proportion of cases? In part, this speaks to popular critiques about 'rational actor' theories in understanding human motivation and agency, but more specifically there is an abundance of evidence regarding the lack of understanding on the part of those targeted by benefit sanctions, which may severely hamper their capacity to comply with relevant behavioural requirements, even if they would wish to (Griggs and Evans, 2010; Wright and Stewart, 2016). Without a plausible theory of change based on available resource and institutional constraints, conditional welfare measures can be considered neither efficacious nor ethical.

Fourth, and following on from the 'in principle' plausibility of the conditional measure, is the question of its *effectiveness in practice*. This must be considered via empirical evidence on whether the specific intervention at issue (or ones like it) can be shown to bring about, or contribute to, the desired behavioural changes – and thereby the ultimate societal goals sought. As discussed above, the evidence on effectiveness is at best mixed on some of the key forms of conditionality, including out-of-work benefit sanctions, though there is more consistent supportive evidence on other conditional measures such as CCTs (Fiszbein et al., 2009) and some anti-social behaviour interventions, for example (Flint, 2011). Equally important, however, is to consider whether the measure may be counterproductive, producing 'scar' effects which generate hostility towards support services, for example (see also Grant, 2006, on the effects on 'character'), or negative spill-over effects, on health, crime, homelessness and so on, that are sufficiently serious to cancel out or even outweigh the benefits of the policy. The sort of comprehensive evidence base required would, ideally, comprise controlled 'pilots' involving quantitative and qualitative research that tracks outcomes over time, and the impacts on wider aspects of people's lives, including giving a strong central place to 'user voice' in understanding the consequences of conditionality. This would allow for a full evaluation of impacts *prior* to programme expansion. If this effectiveness in practice cannot be established, and certainly if there is evidence of counterproductive or spill-over effects that overwhelm any positive benefits, then the conditional welfare programme cannot be considered efficacious or ethical.

Fifth, even if the effectiveness of an overall programme is established, one must still reflect on the '*added value*' of the specific conditional element within it. In other words, why was a non-conditional intervention considered insufficient to achieve the behaviour change and ultimate ends sought? The importance of this question arises from our starting characterisation of conditionality as an exercise of social control. As such, it requires robust ethical justification because of the challenge that it poses both to notions of liberty, given its coercive quality (Lukes, 2005), and also to egalitarian notions of justice, because of the (sometimes) harsh and (often) disproportionate impact on the least well-off in society. Pertinent questions here include: are there alternative, less coercive approaches that can work just as well, and do less coercive approaches tend to be used to achieve similar sorts of behavioural changes with better-off groups? One illustration of this point discussed above relates to CCTs. Though often shown to be effective in meeting their aims, controversy persists over the import of their conditional element, with UCTs and other mechanisms (such as education and the provision of information) shown to be equally or more effective in some instances (Singer, 2015). If no 'added value' can be shown to be associated with the conditional element of a welfare programme, it can be considered neither efficacious nor ethical.

Sixth, even if it is accepted that some degree of conditionality is warranted by the added value that it brings to a welfare programme, a further question relates to the *proportionality* of the specific techniques of conditionality employed. Once again, this arises from the ethical requirement to robustly justify exercises of 'power over' other people, and to limit such exercises to the minimum necessary to achieve the legitimate aims sought. Particularly in the light of the severe hardship evidently caused by some of the harsher benefit sanctioning regimes, this requirement of proportionality might be quite an exacting criterion for some of these programmes to meet. Likewise, the use of strong enforcement measures like Anti-Social Behaviour Orders with street homeless people, which potentially carry long prison sentences, and job-related requirements that demand the equivalent of full-time working hours spent on work search, require strenuous justification on proportionality grounds, i.e. to demonstrate that other less-controlling methods would not be capable of achieving the same results. Otherwise, they fall foul of the criteria for ethical legitimacy, though not necessarily that of effectiveness.

Seventh, and finally, even where it can be demonstrated that a particular conditional welfare intervention achieves its intended and legitimate aims, with zero or minimal unintended negative impacts, the question remains whether these gains are being achieved at the lowest possible *cost*, or at least at an acceptably low cost. The implementation of conditional welfare, and specifically the monitoring and verification processes that are an indispensable feature of conditional programmes, come with a financial cost in terms of administrative infrastructure and staff time, and there are also costs to claimants, both in terms of time spent demonstrating compliance and sometimes in financial terms too. If the same set of outcomes can be achieved at a lower (net) cost, without compromising positive outcomes in relation to the prior questions listed above, then the intervention cannot be considered efficacious. Though this does not *necessarily* impact on the question of its ethical legitimacy, it may well do in the sense that the inflated cost incurred has an opportunity cost in terms of other investments foregone.

It is of course important to emphasise that many of the questions identified above raise matters of judgement and balance, of both an empirical and value-based variety, rather than inviting categorical yes/no answers. This framework is therefore intended as a heuristic device, intended to help systematise the questions that need to be asked and their suggested ordering. By way of summary, we propose asking the following questions of particular examples of conditional welfare interventions in specific contexts:

1. Does this case of behavioural conditionality seek **legitimate ends**, defensible from appropriate and, ideally, multiple normative perspectives?
2. Does the behaviour change incentivised by the proposed conditions **align with the ultimate societal goals** sought?
3. Is the conditional approach underpinned by a **plausible theory of change** regarding the desired impact of the requirements, monitoring mechanisms and threatened sanctions on the behaviour of those targeted?
4. Is there compelling evidence of the **effectiveness in practice** of the conditional approach in bringing about the desired behavioural changes and the ultimate societal goals sought?
5. Does the conditional element of the approach bring **added value**, over and above alternative, non-coercive means of pursuing behavioural change/the goals sought?
6. Are the techniques of conditionality used **proportionate**, i.e. do they deploy the minimum level of 'power over' people commensurate with achieving the relevant goals?
7. Is the conditional intervention **cost-effective** relative to the available alternatives?

As can be seen, questions one to three demand a full interrogation of the ethics and logic of the proposed conditional intervention in principle, and *prior* to any attempt to implement it. In our view, only if compelling answers to these questions can be given is there just cause to progress to implementation. Questions four to seven demand that attempts to design and implement conditional welfare interventions take full heed of existing interventions *and* take seriously the need to fully assess impacts and costs on an ongoing basis and relative to alternative means of achieving the same ends.

It should by now be clear that this proposed analytical framework sets the bar fairly high for welfare conditionality to be considered both effective and ethical, with many evidential and normative 'hoops' to be jumped through before such a conclusion can be soundly reached. That said, it is certainly the case that some instances of welfare conditionality could 'pass' all of the relevant tests. Relevant here are instances in northern Europe of relatively generous benefit systems, offering high replacement rates, in conditions of high employment, and where only relatively mild sanctions (of short duration and/or a low proportion of total benefit income) are imposed for failure to adhere to modest job search activities (Langenbucher, 2015). If the imposition of sanctions in these circumstances leaves those subject to them with all of their basic needs met, and far from destitution, it is difficult to uphold strong moral objections to them, especially if they can be shown to have beneficial incentive effects. In other cases, it is possible that conditionality may not only be ethically permissible, but even ethically required, for example, in those instances of conditionality that demonstrably 'safeguard the future autonomy of people ... facing life-threatening challenges' (Watts et al., 2017, p.13) such as some street homeless people. However, what is equally clear is that the recent intensification of sanctions-backed conditionality in UK out-of-work benefits, far less the much longer-standing and extraordinarily harsh regime in some parts of the US, are a very long distance from meeting the systematic tests set out above.

## Putting conditionality in context

We finish this book where we began, with a consideration of the broader context for welfare conditionality. Conduct requirements are a legitimate source of concern and debate within social policy, in particular where the associated sanctions involve the sorts of brutal impacts on those already experiencing poverty (many of whom are also vulnerable in other ways) reviewed in this book. Whatever the good (or bad) intentions behind such sanctions-backed conditionality, we have argued that it is the *consequences* of such approaches that must be considered paramount. There is clear-enough evidence of the great hardship suffered by those subject to the harsher forms of benefit sanctions that this has to weigh very heavily in any balanced assessment of their merits. The extreme, one might argue disproportionate, nature of some of these penalties, which can be many times more severe than those exacted by the criminal justice system at the more trivial end of the offences spectrum (Webster, 2015a; Adler, 2016), can make a very tall order of attempts to justify them ethically. Such normative concerns are compounded by knowledge of the meagre nature of the infringements that can sometimes provoke sanctions, and the evident lack of intent on the part of many of the claimants who fall foul of relevant requirements (Griggs and Evans, 2010; Wright and Stewart, 2016; Reeve, 2017).

However, it is important for social policy analysts and others not to become so distracted by headline issues of conditionality and sanctions that they neglect the other ethically-relevant dimensions upon which welfare arrangements may vary. Behavioural forms of conditionality, it must always be remembered, are only one form of *targeting*, and not necessarily the most regressive (indeed, as noted above, there are circumstances where conditionality can be supported from a social justice point of view). It is possible for entire impoverished groups to be removed from the 'universe' of applicants eligible for benefits. We have seen this recently in the UK, for example, with the attempt by the Cameron/Osborne-led Conservative administration to remove most people under 22 years of age from entitlement to Housing Benefit. Such an approach is much more 'efficient' for a government intent on driving down welfare budgets, and saves the trouble (and expense) of designing, implementing and monitoring behavioural requirements (National Audit Office, 2016), the meeting of which would then allow the compliant welfare service users to receive relevant benefits or services.

Also critical is the question of whether benefits are received as a matter of legal entitlement or discretion. While there was a lively historical debate about this in the UK – not least between David Donnison (1977) and Richard Titmuss (1958) – there has recently been an insidious shift towards a much more localised, uneven and discretionary welfare safety net, especially in England, with little fanfare or protest (Fitzpatrick et al., 2017). One can see this perhaps most clearly at the housing/welfare interface, with the increasingly heavy reliance on budget-limited Discretionary Housing Payments to meet the shortfall between actual rents and the maximum tenants can receive via the entitlement-based Housing Benefit system. So far the main income maintenance benefits have retained their entitlement status, if not their 'real' monetary value (Beatty and Fothergill, 2016b), but the recent imposition of a (lowered) total benefit cap in particular has radically increased the reliance of affected out-of-work families on discretionary top-ups to enable them to afford any form of accommodation (CIH, 2017). This may be viewed as a politically astute way of eroding the 'rights' basis of UK cash transfer benefits, arousing much less controversy in the mainstream press than the headline-grabbing 'Bedroom Tax' (Meers, 2014) or even benefit sanctions (Adler, 2016).

However, perhaps the most often neglected issue, certainly in contemporary UK debates, is the most basic one of all: their generosity. The understandable focus on matters of structure and principle in the benefits system can distract from the fundamental issue of how much money people are given to live on. The ongoing freeze in working-age benefits in the UK is by far the most important element in the £12 billion worth of further savings in welfare spend planned during this Parliament (Department for Work Pensions, 2015), and is consequently a pre-eminent factor in the rise in UK child poverty predicted to occur between now and 2021/22, which will affect the North East of England and Wales worst of all (Hood and Waters, 2017a).

What seems particularly difficult to justify from any plausible ethical perspective is to pay cash transfer benefits at such a very low level that even those who are in theory protected by the welfare safety net are in reality left destitute. It was estimated that 1.25 million people in the UK experienced destitution at some point in 2015, the great majority of them UK citizens (Fitzpatrick et al., 2016). While benefit sanctions played an important role in a substantial number of these cases, even more important was that rates of working-age benefits are now so meagre that people getting by on these minimal allowances for any length of time are very easily tipped into absolute destitution. With growing evidence that poverty is costly for society as a whole (Bramley et al., 2015; Joseph Rowntree Foundation, 2016), as well as being profoundly harmful for those directly affected by it (Pemberton et al., 2018), UK welfare policies which are predicted to drive it up in the coming years look to be neither efficacious nor ethical.

Thus, in the UK at least, there is an important wider context within which to place anxieties about welfare conditionality. Our concern about its deleterious impacts, or indeed our hopes with regard to its benefits, cannot be allowed to eclipse our judgement about the wider welfare context within which such measures sit. Some of the most conditional welfare systems (notably, in Scandinavia) are also the most generous, for those who manage to meet stringent behavioural and other requirements. Indeed, an explicit trade-off between conditionality (and other forms of targeting) and generosity can often be seen in welfare policies, which in turn will be determined by ideological preferences, political priorities and/or embedded societal values (Fitzpatrick and Stephens, 2014).

More broadly, we hope to have demonstrated in this book that sanctions-backed forms of welfare differ enormously in their origins, intentions, implementation and impacts. A universal, 'one-size-fits-all' answer on the questions of whether conditionality 'works' and/or is 'morally justified' is therefore neither possible nor desirable. However, it is possible, we would argue, to deconstruct instances of conditionality into their component parts for detailed empirical and normative scrutiny and come to a view which is properly evidenced, logically consistent and ethically-informed. One might even go so far as to hope that, bolstered by this sort of systematic analysis, a broader consensus may be reached on the desirability of specific conditional approaches, informing the development of evolving welfare systems across the Global North and South.

# BIBLIOGRAPHY

Adler, M. (2016). A new leviathan: Benefit sanctions in the twenty-first century. *Journal of Law and Society*, 43(2), 195–227.

Adler, M. and Terum, L. I. (2017). Austerity, conditionality and the rule of law, in Civitarese Matteucci, S. and Halliday, S. (eds) *Social Rights in Europe in an Age of Austerity*, 147–178. Abingdon: Routledge.

Aldridge, R. W., Story, A., Hwang, S. W., Nordentoft, M., Luchenski, S. A., Hartwell, G., Tweed, E., Lewer, D., Katikireddi, S. V. and Hayward, A. C. (2017). Morbidity and mortality in homeless individuals, prisoners, sex workers, and individuals with substance use disorders in high-income countries: A systematic review and meta-analysis. *The Lancet*. DOI:10.1016/S0140-6736 (17)31869-X

Allen, M. (2012). Quality standards in homeless services, housing led approaches and the legacy of 'Less Eligibility'. *European Journal of Homelessness*, 6(2), 159–166.

Amster, R. (2003). Patterns of exclusion: Sanitising space, criminalising homelessness. *Social Justice*, 30, 195–221.

ANAO (Australian National Audit Office). (2014). *The Improving School Enrolment and Attendance through Welfare Reform Measure, Audit Report No. 51, 2013–14, Performance Audit*. Canberra: ANAO.

Andersen, J. G. (2007). Restricting access to social protection for immigrants in the Danish welfare state. *Benefits*, 15(3), 257–269.

Apps, P. (2016). Government scraps compulsory Pay to Stay. *Inside Housing*, 21st November. www.insidehousing.co.uk/home/home/government-scraps-compulsory-pay-to-stay-48717

Arni, P., Lalive, R. and van Ours, J. (2009). *How Effective are Unemployment Benefit Sanctions? Looking Beyond Unemployment Exit. IZA Discussion Paper No. 4509*. Bonn: Institute for the Study of Labor (IZA).

Attoh, K. A. (2011). What kind of right is the right to the city? *Progress in Human Geography*, 35(5), 669–685.

Australian Government. (2009). *Policy Statement: Landmark Reform to the Welfare System, Reinstatement of the Racial Discrimination Act and Strengthening of the Northern Territory Emergency Response*. Canberra: Australian Government.

Australian Government. (2015). Budget 2015: Growing jobs and small business. www.budget.gov.au/2015-16/content/glossy/sml_bus/download/Growing_Jobs_and_Small_Business.pdf

Australian Public Service Commission. (2007). *Changing Behaviour: A Public Policy Perspective*. Canberra: Australian Government.

Bachrach, P. and Baratz, M. S. (1963). Decisions and non-decisions: An analytical framework. *American Political Science Review*, 57, 641–651.

Bagguley, P. and Mann, K. (1992). Idle thieving bastards? Scholarly representations of the underclass. *Work, Employment and Society*, 6(1), 113–126.

Bailey, N. (2018). Employment, poverty and social exclusion, in Bramley, G. and Bailey, N. (eds) *Poverty and Social Exclusion in the UK. Volume 2 – the Dimensions of Disadvantage*, 159–178. Bristol: Policy Press.

Baird, S., Ferreira, F., Özler, B. and Woolcock, M. (2014). Conditional, unconditional and everything in between: A systematic review of the effects of cash transfer programmes on schooling outcomes. *Journal of Development Effectiveness*, 6(1), 1–43.

Baldwin, D. A. (1971). The power of positive sanctions. *World Politics*, 24(1), 19–38.

Bambra, C. (2007). Going beyond the three worlds of welfare capitalism: Regime theory and public health research. *Journal of Epidemiology and Community Health*, 61(12), 1098–1102.

Barnes, M. and Prior, D. (eds) (2009). *Subversive Citizens: Power, Agency and Resistance in Public Services*. Bristol: Policy Press.

Barnes, S. (2016). Applicants barred by local connection rules. *Inside Housing*, 11th March. www.insidehousing.co.uk/news/news/applicants-barred-by-local-connection-rules-46435

Barr, B., Taylor-Robinson, D., Stuckler, D., Loopstra, R., Reeves, A., Wickham, S. and Whitehead, M. (2016). Fit-for-work or fit-for-unemployment? Does the reassessment of disability benefit claimants using a tougher work capability assessment help people into work? *Journal of Epidemiology and Community Health*, 70(5), 452–458.

Barrientos, A. (2011). Conditions in antipoverty programmes. *Journal of Poverty and Social Justice*, 19(1), 15–26.

Bastagli, F. (2009). Conditionality in public policy targeted to the poor: Promoting resilience? *Social Policy and Society*, 8(1), 127–140.

Batty, E. and Flint, J. (2012). Conceptualising the contexts, mechanisms and outcomes of intensive family intervention projects. *Social Policy and Society*, 11(3), 345–358.

Batty, E., Beatty, C., Casey, R., Foden, M., McCarthy, L. and Reeve, K. (2015). *Homeless People's Experiences of Welfare Conditionality and Benefit Sanctions*. London: Crisis.

Bauman, Z. (1993). *Postmodern Ethics*. Oxford: Blackwell.

Baumberg, B., Warren, J., Garthwaite, K. and Bambra, C. (2015). *Rethinking the Work Capability Assessment*. London: DEMOS.

Bavier, R. (2001). Welfare reform data from the survey of income and program participation. *Monthly Labour Review*, 124, 13–24.

Beatty, C. and Fothergill, S. (2013). *Hitting the Poorest Places Hardest: The Local and Regional Impact of Welfare Reform*. Sheffield: CRESR, Sheffield Hallam University.

Beatty, C. and Fothergill, S. (2016a). *Jobs, Welfare and Austerity: How the Destruction of Industrial Britain Casts a Shadow Over Present-day Public Finances*. Sheffield: CRESR, Sheffield Hallam University.

Beatty, C. and Fothergill, S. (2016b). *The Uneven Impact of Welfare Reform: The Financial Losses to Places and People*. Sheffield: CRESR, Sheffield Hallam University.

Bell, D. N. and Blanchflower, D. G. (2011). Young people and the great recession. *Oxford Review of Economic Policy*, 27(2), 241–267.

Bellis, M. A., Lowey, H., Leckenby, N., Hughes, K. and Harrison, D. (2014). Adverse childhood experiences: Retrospective study to determine their impact on adult health behaviours and health outcomes in a UK population. *Journal of Public Health*, 36(1), 81–91.

Bengtsson, B. (2001). Housing as a social right: Implications for welfare state theory. *Scandinavian Political Studies*, 24(4), 255–275.

Bentham, J. (1791/1995). *The Panopticon Writings. Introduction by Miran Božovič*. New York, NY: Verso.

Berlin, I. (1969). *Four Essays on Liberty*. Oxford: Oxford University Press.

Bertrand, M., Mullainathan, S. and Shafir, E. (2004). A behavioral-economics view of poverty. *American Economic Review*, 94(2), 419–423.

Beveridge, W. (1942). *Social Insurance and Allied Services*. London: Her Majesty's Stationery Office.

Bhukuth, A. and Ballet, J. (2015). Children of the street: Why are they in the street? How do they live? *Economics and Sociology*, 8(4), 134–148.

Bielefeld, S. (2012). Compulsory income management and Indigenous Australians: Delivering social justice or furthering colonial domination. *University of New South Wales Law Journal*, 35(2), 522–562.

Black, C. (2016). *An Independent Review into the Impact on Employment Outcomes of Drug or Alcohol Addiction, and Obesity*. London: Her Majesty's Stationery Office.

Bonjour, D., Dorsett, R., Knight, G., Lissenburgh, S., Mukherjee, A., Payne, J., Range, M., Urwin, P. and White, M. (2001). *New Deal for Young People: National Survey of Participants: Stage 2, Employment Service Research and Development Report*. Sheffield: Employment Service.

Bonoli, B. (2010). *The Political Economy of Active Labour Market Policy. REC-WP 01/2010 Working Papers on the Reconciliation of Work and Welfare in Europe*. Edinburgh: Dissemination and Dialogue Centre.

Bothfeld, S. and Rosenthal, P. (2017). The end of social security as we know it: The erosion of status protection in German labour market policy. *Journal of Social Policy*, 1–20. DOI:10.1017/S0047279417000332

Bowpitt, G., Dwyer, P., Sundin, E. and Weinstein, M. (2014). Places of sanctuary for 'the undeserving'? Homeless people's day centres and the problem of conditionality. *British Journal of Social Work*, 44(5), 1251–1267.

Brady, D., Fullerton, A. S. and Cross, J. M. (2009). Putting poverty in political context: A multi-level analysis of adult poverty across 18 affluent democracies. *Social Forces*, 88(1), 271–299.

Bramley, G. and Bailey, N. (eds) (2018). *Poverty and Social Exclusion in the UK. Volume 2 – The Dimensions of Disadvantage*. Bristol: Policy Press.

Bramley, G. and Fitzpatrick, S. (2017). Homelessness in the UK: Who is most at risk? *Housing Studies*, 33(1), 96–116.

Bramley, G., Fitzpatrick, S., Edwards, J., Ford, D., Johnsen, S., Sosenko, F. and Watkins, D. (2015) *Hard Edges: Mapping Severe and Multiple Disadvantage*. London: Lankelly Chase Foundation.

Bramley, G., Hirsch, D., Littlewood, M. and Watkins, D. (2016). *Counting the Cost of UK Poverty*. York: Joseph Rowntree Foundation.

Bray, J. R., Gray, M., Hand, K. and Katz, I. (2014). *Evaluating New Income Management in the Northern Territory: Final Evaluation Report*. Sydney: Social Policy Research Centre, University of New South Wales.

Bretherton, J., Hunter, C. and Johnsen, S. (2013). 'You can judge them on how they look . . .': Homelessness officers, medical evidence and decision-making in England. *European Journal of Homelessness*, 7(1), 69–92.

Brigham, J. and Brown, D. W. (1980). Introduction: Distinguishing penalties and incentives, in Brigham, J. and Brown, D. W. (eds) *Policy Implementation: Penalties or Incentives?* 5–10. Thousand Oaks, CA: Sage.

Brodkin, E. Z. (1997). Inside the welfare contract: Discretion and accountability in state welfare administration. *Social Service Review*, 71(1), 1–33.

Brodkin, E. Z. (2013). Street-level organisations and the welfare state, in Brodkin, E. Z. and Marston, G. (eds) *Work and the Welfare State: Street-level Organizations and Workfare Politics*, 17–34. Washington, DC: Georgetown University Press.

Brodkin, E. Z. and Larsen, F. (2013). The policies of workfare: At the boundaries between work and the welfare state, in Brodkin, E. Z. and Marston, G. (eds) *Work and the Welfare State: Street-level Organizations and Workfare Politics*, 57–67. Washington, DC: Georgetown University Press.

Brown, K. (2016). *Vulnerability and Young People: Care and Social Control in Policy and Practice*. Bristol: Policy Press.

Buckingham, H. (2011). Hybridity, diversity and the division of labour in the third sector: What can we learn from homelessness organisations in the UK? *Voluntary Sector Review*, 2(2), 157–175.

Busch-Geertsema, V. (2014). Housing first Europe: Results of a European social experimentation project. *European Journal of Homelessness*, 8(1), 13–28.

Bywaters, P., Bunting, L., Davidson, G., Hanratty, J., Mason, W., McCartan, C. and Steils, N. (2016). *The Relationship Between Poverty, Child Abuse and Neglect: An Evidence Review*. York: Joseph Rowntree Foundation.

Cabinet Office. (2015). Hancock: Every young person should be earning or learning from April 2017. Cabinet Office press release, 17th August. www.gov.uk/government/news/hancock-every-young-person-should-be-earning-or-learning-from-april-2017

Cabinet Office/Institute for Government. (2010). *MINDSPACE: Influencing Behaviour Through Public Policy*. London: Cabinet Office.

Cain, R. (2016). Responsibilising recovery: Lone and low-paid parents, Universal Credit and the gendered contradictions of UK welfare reform. *British Politics*, 11(4), 488–507.

Caldés, N., Coady, D. and Maluccio, J. A. (2006). The cost of poverty alleviation transfer programs: A comparative analysis of three programs in Latin America. *World Development*, 34(5), 818–837.

Campbell, T., Ewing, K. D. and Tomkins, A. (2011). *The Legal Protection of Human Rights: Sceptical Essays*. Oxford: Oxford University Press.

Caplan, A. (2008). Denying autonomy in order to create it: The paradox of forcing treatment upon addicts. *Addiction*, 103(12), 1919–1921.

Casey, T. (2010). *The Sanction Epidemic in the Temporary Assistance for Needy Families Program*. New York, NY: Legal Momentum, the Women's Legal Defense and Education Fund.

Centre for Social Justice. (2009). *Dying to Belong: An In-depth Review of Street Gangs in Britain*. London: Centre for Social Justice.

Centre for Social Justice. (2013). *Fractured Families: Why Stability Matters*. London: Centre for Social Justice.

Child Welfare League of America. (2017). The President's fiscal year 2018 budget request. www.cwla.org/wp-content/uploads/2017/05/CWLA-Summary-of-Presidents-FY-2018-Childrens-Child-Welfare-Budget.pdf

Chrisafis, A. (2017). Housing benefit cuts spark row as Emmanuel Macron's poll ratings fall. *The Guardian*, 24th July. www.theguardian.com/world/2017/jul/24/housing-benefit-cuts-add-to-fall-in-emmanuel-macrons-popularity

Chriss, J. J. (2007). *Social Control: An Introduction*. Cambridge: Polity Press.

Church Poverty Action Group, Baptist Union of Great Britain, United Reformed Church, Methodist Church, Church of Scotland and Church in Wales. (2015). Time to rethink benefit sanctions. www.jointpublicissues.org.uk/wp-content/uploads/rethink-sanctions-report-0315.pdf

CIH. (2017). Feeling the pinch: The lowered benefit cap one year on. www.cih.org/publication-free/display/vpathDCR/templatedata/cih/publication-free/data/Feeling_the_pinch_the_lowered_benefit_cap_one_year_on

Clarke, J. (2004). *Changing Welfare, Changing States: New Directions in Social Policy*. London: Sage.

Clasen, J. and Clegg, D. (2006). Beyond activation: Reforming European unemployment protection systems in post-industrial labour markets. *European Societies*, 8(4), 527–553.

Clasen, J. and Clegg, D. (2007). Levels and levers of conditionality: Measuring change within welfare states, in Clasen, J. and Siegel, N. A. (eds) *The 'Dependent Variable Problem' in Comparative Analysis*, 166–197. Cheltenham: Edward Elgar.

Coleman, A. (2000). Five-star motels: Spaces, places and homelessness in Fortitude Valley, Brisbane. Unpublished PhD thesis. St Lucia: University of Queensland.

Conservative Home. (2012). Many councils oppose housing policies that reward work, volunteering, and service in the armed forces. *Conservative Home*, 13th August. www.conservativehome.com/localgovernment/2012/08/many-councils-opposing-housing-policies-to-reward-work-volunteering-and-service-in-the-armed-forces.html

Cowan, D. (2011). *Housing Law and Policy*. Cambridge: Cambridge University Press.

Crisp, R. and Fletcher, D. R. (2008). *A Comparative Review of Workfare Programmes in the United States, Canada and Australia (No. 533)*. London: Department for Work and Pensions.

Curchin, K. (2017). Using behavioural insights to argue for a stronger social safety net: Beyond libertarian paternalism. *Journal of Social Policy*, 46(2), 231–249.

Daguerre, A. (2008). The second phase of US welfare reform, 2000–2006: Blaming the poor again? *Social Policy and Administration*, 42(4), 362–378.

Daguerre, A. (2013). The new frontiers of welfare reform under the presidency of Barack Obama. Congrès Association Francaise de Science Politique, 6th July, Paris. http://workfare.org.uk/images/uploads/docs/st1daguerre.pdf

Daguerre, A. and Etherington, D. (2014). *Workfare in 21st Century Britain: The Erosion of Rights to Social Assistance*. London: Middlesex University.

Dahrendorf, R. (1987). The underclass and the future of Britain. Paper presented at the 10th Annual Lecture, Windsor: St George's House.

Dar, A. (2016). Help to work: Post-work programme provision for the long-term unemployed. House of Commons Library Briefing Paper Number 6904. http://researchbriefings.parliament.uk/ResearchBriefing/Summary/SN06904#fullreport

Darnton, A. (2008). GSR Behaviour Change Knowledge Review – reference report: An overview of behaviour change models and their uses. Government Social Research.

Dawnay, E. and Shah, H. (2005). *Behavioural Economics: 7 Principles for Policy-makers*. London: New Economics Foundation.

DCLG. (2010). *Local Decisions: A Fairer Future for Social Housing*. London: DCLG.

DCLG. (2012). *Allocation of Accommodation: Guidance for Local Housing Authorities in England*. London: DCLG.

DCLG. (2016). *Lifetime Tenancies: Equality Impact Assessment*. London: DCLG.

De Agostini, P., Hills, J. and Sutherland, S. (2014). *Were We Really All in it Together? The Distributional Effects of the UK Coalition Government's Tax-benefit Policy Changes. CASE: Working Paper 10*. London: London School of Economics and Political Science.

De Decker, P. (2009). Social rental agencies: Still a splendid idea? *European Journal of Homelessness*, 3, 217–232.

de Vries, R., Reeves, B. and Baumberg-Geiger, B. (2017). *Inequalities in the Application of Welfare Sanctions in Britain: Working Paper 15*. London: London School of Economics.

Deacon, A. (1994). Justifying workfare: The historical context of the workfare debates, in White, M. (ed) *Unemployment and Public Policy in a Changing Labour Market*, 53–63. London: Policy Studies Institute.

Deacon, A. (2004). Justifying conditionality: The case of anti-social tenants. *Housing Studies*, 19(6), 911–926.

Deacon, A. and Mann, K. (1999). Agency, modernity and social policy. *Journal of Social Policy*, 28(3), 413–435.

Dean, H. (1991). *Social Security and Social Control*. London: Routledge.

Dean, M. (1991). *The Constitution of Poverty: Toward a Genealogy of Liberal Governance*. Abingdon: Routledge.

Dean, H. (2002). *Welfare Rights and Social Policy*. Harlow: Pearson Education.

Dean, H. (ed). (2004). *The Ethics of Welfare: Human Rights, Dependency and Responsibility*. Bristol: Policy Press.

Dean, H. (2010). *Understanding Human Need*. Bristol: Policy Press.

Dean, H. and Taylor-Gooby, P. (1992). *Dependency Culture: The Explosion of a Myth*. London: Harvester Wheatsheaf.

Deci, E. L. and Ryan, R. M. (2008). Self-determination theory: A macrotheory of human motivation, development, and health. *Canadian psychology/Psychologie canadienne*, 49(3), 182.

Dennis, N. (1993). *Rising Crime and the Dismembered Family: How Conformist Intellectuals have Campaigned Against Common Sense*. London: IEA Health and Welfare Unit.

Dennis, N. and Erdos, G. (1992). *Families Without Fathers*. London: Institute of Economic Affairs.

Department for Work and Pensions. (2015). *An Independent Review into the Impact on Employment Outcomes of Drug or Alcohol Addiction, and Obesity: Call for Evidence*. London: DWP.

Department for Work and Pensions. (2016). JSA sanctions early warning trial evaluation – Interim report. www.gov.uk/government/uploads/system/uploads/attachment_data/file/578691/jobseekers-allowance-sanctions-early-warning-trial-evaluation-interim-report.pdf

Devany, C. (2017). Youth unemployment, welfare stigmatization and mental health. Housing Studies Association blog, 7th December. http://housing-studies-association.org/2017/12/blog-youth-unemployment-welfare-stigma tization-mental-health/

DeVerteuil, G. (2014). Does the punitive need the supportive? A sympathetic critique of current grammars of urban injustice. *Antipode*, 46(4), 874–893.

Deverteuil, G., May, J. and von Mahs, J. (2009). Complexity not collapse: Recasting the geographies of homelessness in a 'punitive' age. *Progress in Human Geography*, 33(5), 646–666.

Dewar, L. and Ben-Galim, D. (2017). *An Impossible Bind: Requirements to Work Under Universal Credit*. London: Gingerbread.

Dhaliwal, I., Duflo, E., Glennerster, R. and Tulloch, C. (2014). Comparative cost-effectiveness analysis to inform policy in developing countries: A general framework with applications for education, in Glewwe, P. (ed) *Education Policy in Developing Countries*, 285–338. Chicago, IL: University of Chicago Press.

Digby, A. (1989). *British Welfare Policy: Workhouse to Workfare*. London: Faber and Faber.

Doherty, J., Busch-Geertsema, V., Karpuskiene, V., Korhonen, J., O'Sullivan, E., Sahlin, I., Tosi, A., Petrillo, A. and Wygnanska, J. (2008). Homelessness and exclusion: Regulating public space in European cities. *Surveillance and Society*, 5(3), 290–314.

Dolan, P., Hallsworth, M., Halpern, D., King, D., Metcalfe, R. and Vlaev, I. (2012). Influencing behaviour: The mindspace way. *Journal of Economic Psychology*, 33(1), 264–277.

Donnison, D. (1977). Against discretion. *New Society*, 41, 534–536.

Dorsett, R. (2008). *Pathways to Work for New and Repeat Incapacity Benefits claimants: Evaluation Synthesis Report, Department for Work and Pensions. Research Report No. 525.* Norwich: Her Majesty's Stationery Office.

Doyal, L. and I. Gough. (1991). *A Theory of Human Need*. Basingstoke: Palgrave Macmillan.

Duncan-Smith, I. (2006). *Breakdown Britain: Interim Report on the State of the Nation*. London: Centre for Social Justice.

Dunn, A. (2014). *Rethinking Unemployment and the Work Ethic: Beyond the 'Quasi-Titmuss' Paradigm*. Basingstoke: Palgrave MacMillan.

Durkheim, E. (1893/1984). *The Division of Labor in Society*. Trans. W. D. Halls. New York, NY: Free Press.

Dwelly, T. and Cowans, J. (2006). *Rethinking Social Housing*. London: Smith Institute.

Dworkin, R. (1977). *Taking Rights Seriously*. London: Duckworth.

Dworkin, R. (2000). *Sovereign Virtue: The Theory and Practice of Equality*. Cambridge, MA: Harvard University Press.

Dwyer, P. (1998). Conditional citizens? Welfare rights and responsibilities in the late 1990's. *Critical Social Policy*, 18(4), 519–543.

Dwyer, P. (2000). *Welfare Rights and Responsibilities: Contesting Social Citizenship*. Bristol: Policy Press.

Dwyer, P. (2004). Creeping conditionality in the UK: From welfare rights to conditional entitlements. *Canadian Journal or Sociology*, 29(2), 265–287.

Dwyer, P. (2009). *Integration? The Perceptions and Experiences of Refugees in Yorkshire and the Humber*. Leeds: Yorkshire and Humber Regional Migration Partnership.

Dwyer, P. (2010). *Understanding Social Citizenship: Themes and Perspectives for Policy and Practice*. Bristol: Policy Press.

Dwyer, P. (2016). *Context Briefing: Migrants. Welfare Conditionality: Sanctions, Support and Behaviour Change*. York: University of York.

Dwyer, P. and Bright, J. (2016). *First Wave Findings: Overview. Welfare Conditionality: Sanctions, Support and Behaviour Change*. York: University of York.

Dwyer, P. and Wright, S. (2014). Universal credit, ubiquitous conditionality and its implications for social citizenship. *Journal of Poverty and Social Justice*, 22(1), 27–35.

Dwyer, P., Jones, K., McNeill, J., Scullion, L. and Stewart, A. (2016). *Welfare Conditionality: Sanctions, Support and Behaviour Change*. York: University of York.

Eichhorst, W. and Konle-Seidl, R. (2008). *Contingent Convergence: A Comparative Analysis of Activation Policies*. Bonn: Institute for the Study of Labour.

Elster, J. (1983). *Sour Grapes: Studies in the Subversion of Rationality*. Cambridge: Cambridge University Press.

Epel, E. S., Bandura, A. and Zimbardo, P. G. (1999). Escaping homelessness: The influences of self-efficacy and time perspective on coping with homelessness. *Journal of Applied Social Psychology*, 29(3), 575–596.

Esping-Andersen, G. (1990). *The Three Worlds of Welfare Capitalism*. Cambridge: Polity Press.

Etzioni, A. (1994). *The Politics of Community*. London: Fontana.

Etzioni, A. (1997). *The New Golden Rule*. London: Profile Books.

Etzioni, A. (ed) (1998). *The Essential Communitarian Reader*. Oxford: Rowman and Littlefield.

EUROCEF. (2012). Truancy and suspensions allocs. What about the Council of Europe? *EUROCEF*, 18th December. http://eurocef.eu/en/suspensions-allowances-council-of-europe

Eurofound. (2016). *Inadequate Housing in Europe: Costs and Consequences*. Luxembourg: Publications Office of the European Union.

European Commission. (2014). *Study on Conditional Cash Transfers and their Impact on Children*. Brussels: European Commission.

Evans, T. (2016). *Professional Discretion in Welfare Services: Beyond Street-level Bureaucracy*. Abingdon: Routledge.

Fahmy, E., Williamson, E. and Pantazis, C. (2016). *Evidence and Policy Review: Domestic Violence and Poverty*. York: Joseph Rowntree Foundation.

Falk, G. (2016). *Temporary Assistance for Needy Families (TANF): Size and Characteristics of the Cash Assistance Caseload*. Washington, DC: Congressional Research Service.

Falk, G., McCarty, M. and Aussenberg, R. A. (2014). *Work Requirements, Time Limits, and Work Incentives in TANF, SNAP, and Housing Assistance*. Washington, DC: Congressional Research Service.

Farnsworth, K. and Irving, Z. M. (eds) (2011). *Social Policy in Challenging Times: Economic Crisis and Welfare Systems*. Bristol: Policy Press.

Fernald, L. C., Gertler, P. J. and Neufeld, L. M. (2008). Role of cash in conditional cash transfer programmes for child health, growth, and development: An analysis of Mexico's Oportunidades. *The Lancet*, 371(9615), 828–837.

Fernandez Evangelista, G. and Jones, S. (2013). *Mean Streets: A Report on the Criminalization of Homelessness in Europe*. Brussels: FEANTSA.

Field, F. (1989). *Losing Out: The Emergence of Britain's Underclass*. Oxford: Blackwell.

Finch, J. D. (1979). *Introduction to Legal Theory*. London: Sweet & Maxwell.

Finn, D. and Gloster, R. (2010). *Lone Parent Obligations: A Review of Recent Evidence on the Work-related Requirements within the Benefit Systems of Different Countries*. London: DWP.

Finn, D. and Goodship, J. (2014). *Take-up of Benefits and Poverty: An Evidence and Policy Review*. London: Centre for Economic and Social Inclusion.

Fiszbein, A., Schady, N. R. with Ferreira, F., Grosh, M., Keleher, N., Olinto, P. and Skoufias, E. (2009). *Conditional Cash Transfers: Reducing Present and Future Poverty*. Washington, DC: World Bank.

Fitzpatrick, S. and Johnsen, S. (2009). The use of enforcement to combat 'street culture' in England: An ethical approach? *Ethics and Social Welfare*, 3(3), 284–302.

Fitzpatrick, S. and Pawson, H. (2011). *Security of Tenure in Social Housing: An International Review*. London: Shelter.

Fitzpatrick, S. and Pawson, H. (2014). Ending security of tenure for social renters: Transitioning to 'ambulance service' social housing? *Housing Studies*, 29(5), 597–615.

Fitzpatrick, S. and Pawson, H. (2016). Fifty years since *Cathy Come Home*: Critical reflections on the UK homelessness safety net. *International Journal of Housing Policy*, 16(4), 543–555.

Fitzpatrick, S. and Stephens, M. (1999). Homelessness, need and desert in the allocation of council housing. *Housing Studies*, 14(4), 413–431.

Fitzpatrick, S. and Stephens, M. (2007). *An International Review of Homelessness and Social Housing Policy*. London: Communities and Local Government.

Fitzpatrick, S. and Stephens, M. (2014). Welfare regimes, social values and homelessness: Comparing responses to marginalised groups in six European countries. *Housing Studies*, 29(2), 215–234.

Fitzpatrick, S. and Watts, B. (2016). Poverty and complex needs, in Joseph Rowntree Foundation (ed) *UK Poverty: Causes, Costs and Solutions*, 217–247. York: Joseph Rowntree Foundation.

Fitzpatrick, S. and Watts, B. (2017). Competing visions: Security of tenure and the welfarisation of English social housing. *Housing Studies*, 32(8), 1021–1038.

Fitzpatrick, S., Bengtsson, B. and Watts, B. (2014). Rights to housing: Reviewing the terrain and exploring a way forward. *Housing, Theory and Society*, 31(4), 447–463.

Fitzpatrick, S., Bramley, G., Sosenko, F., Blenkinsopp, J., Johnsen, S., Littlewood, M., Netto, G. and Watts, B. (2016). *Destitution in the UK*. York: Joseph Rowntree Foundation.

Fitzpatrick, S., Kennedy, C., Kintrea, K. and Mullen, T. (2002). *Social Justice Committee 3rd Report 2002: Monitoring the Impact of the Housing (Scotland). Act 2001*. Edinburgh: Scottish Parliament.

Fitzpatrick, S., Pawson, H., Bramley, G., Wilcox, S. and Watts, B. (2015). *The Homelessness Monitor: Wales 2015*. London: Crisis.

Fitzpatrick, S., Pawson, H., Bramley, G., Wilcox, S. and Watts, B. (2017). *The Homelessness Monitor: England 2017*. London: Crisis.

Fletcher, D. R. (2008). Offenders in the post-industrial labour market: From the underclass to the undercaste? *Policy & Politics*, 26(2), 283–297.

Fletcher, D. R. (2013). The governance of social marginality in the UK: Towards the centaur state? *British Journal of Community Justice*, 11(1), 19–34.

Fletcher, D. R. and Wright, S. (2017). A hand up or a slap down? Criminalising benefit claimants in Britain via strategies of surveillance, sanctions and deterrence. *Critical Social Policy*, DOI: 10.1177/0261018317726622.

Fletcher, D. R., Flint, J., Batty, E. and McNeill, J. (2016). Gamers or victims of the system? Welfare reform, cynical manipulation and vulnerability. *Journal of Poverty and Social Justice*, 24(2), 171–185.

Flint, C. (2008). Address to Fabian Society, Future of Housing Conference, London, February 5.

Flint, J. (2002). Return of the governors: Citizenship and the new governance of neighbourhood disorder in the UK. *Citizenship Studies*, 6(3), 245–264.

Flint J. (2006). Housing and the new governance of conduct, in Flint, J. (ed) *Housing, Urban Governance and Anti-social Behaviour Perspectives, Policy and Practice*, 19–36. Bristol: Policy Press.

Flint, J. (2009a). Governing marginalised populations: The role of coercion, support and agency. *European Journal of Homelessness*, 3, 247–260.

Flint, J. (2009b). Subversive subjects and conditional, earned and denied citizenship, in Barnes, M. and Prior, D. (eds) *Subversive Citizens: Power, Agency and Resistance in Public Services*, 83–98. Bristol: Policy Press.

Flint, J. (2011). The role of sanctions in intensive support and rehabilitation: Rhetoric, rationalities and realities. *British Journal of Community Justice*, 9(1/2), 55–67.

Flint, J. (2012). The inspection house and neglected dynamics of governance: The case of domestic visits in family intervention projects. *Housing Studies*, 27(6), 822–838.

Flint, J. (2015). Housing and the realignment of urban socio-spatial contracts. *Housing, Theory and Society*, 32(1), 39–53.

Flint, J. (forthcoming). Encounters with the centaur state: Advanced urban marginality and the practices and ethics of welfare sanctions regimes. *Urban Studies*.

Flint, J. and Nixon, J. (2006). Governing neighbours: Anti-social behaviour orders and new forms of regulating conduct in the UK. *Urban Studies*, 43 (5–6), 939–955.

Flint, J., Jones, A. and Parr, S. (2011). *An Evaluation of the Sanction of Housing Benefit*. London: DWP.

Fording, R. C., Schram, S. F. and Soss, J. (2013). Do welfare sanctions help or hurt the poor? Estimating the causal effect of sanctioning on client earnings. *Social Service Review*, 87(4), 641–676.

Fortman, B. (2006). Poverty as a failure of entitlement: Do rights-based approaches make sense? in Williams, L. (ed) *International Poverty Law: An Emerging Discourse*, 34–48. London: Zed Books.

Foster, D. (2016). Adam Perkins: 'Welfare dependency can be bred out'. *The Guardian*, 9th March. www.theguardian.com/society/2016/mar/09/adam-perkins-welfare-dependency-can-be-bred-out

Fouarge, D. and Layte, R. (2005). Welfare regimes and poverty dynamics: The duration and recurrence of poverty spells in Europe. *Journal of Social Policy*, 34 (3), 407–426.

Freeland, N. (2007). Superfluous, pernicious, atrocious and abominable? The case against conditional cash transfers. *IDS Bulletin*, 38(3), 75–78.

Freud, D. (2007). *Reducing Dependency, Increasing Opportunity: Options for the Future of Welfare to Work*. London: DWP.

Friedli, L. and Stearn, R. (2015). Positive affect as coercive strategy: Conditionality, activation and the role of psychology in UK government workfare programmes. *Medical Humanities*, 41(1), 40–47.

Frost, N. A. (2010). Beyond public opinion polls: Punitive public sentiment and criminal justice policy. *Sociology Compass*, 4(3), 156–168.

Gabriel, I. (2017). Effective altruism and its critics. *Journal of Applied Philosophy*, 34(4), 457–473.

Garthwaite, K. (2016). *Hunger Pains: Life Inside Foodbank Britain*. Bristol: Policy Press.

Garvie, D. (2012). *Local Decisions on Tenure Reform. Local Tenancy Strategies and the New Role of Local Housing Authorities in Leading Tenure Policy*. London: Shelter.

Geiger, B. B. (2012). The mysterious non-claiming unemployed. Inequalities Blog, 9th March. https://inequalitiesblog.wordpress.com/2012/03/09/the-mysterious-non-claiming-unemloyed/

Geiger, B. B. (2017). Benefits conditionality for disabled people: Stylized facts from a review of international evidence and practice. *Journal of Poverty and Social Justice*, 25(2), 107–128.

Gibb, K. (2012). Behavioural economics, in Smith, S. J. (ed) *International Encyclopedia of Housing and Home*, Vol. 1, 97–102. Amsterdam: Elsevier.

Goodin, R. E. (1985). *Protecting the Vulnerable: A Re-Analysis of Our Social Responsibilities*. Chicago, IL/London: University of Chicago Press.

Goodin, R. E. (1986). Welfare, rights and discretion. *Oxford Journal of Legal Studies*, 6(2), 232–261.

Goodin, R. E. (1993). Utility and the good, in Singer, P. (ed) *A Companian to Ethics*, 241–248. Oxford: Blackwell.

Goodin, R. E. (2002). Structures of mutual obligation. *Journal of Social Policy*, 31 (4), 579–596.

Goodwin, T. (2012). Why we should reject 'nudge'. *Politics*, 32(2), 85–92.

Goodwin, V. (2008). *The Effects of Benefit Sanctions on Lone Parents' Employment Decisions and Moves into Employment. DWP Research Report No. 511*. Norwich: Her Majesty's Stationery Office.

Gordon, R. (2008). What is Housing First and supportive housing? *Parity*, 21, 4–5.

Gough, I. (1998). What are human needs? in Franklin, J. (ed) *Social Policy and Social Work: The IPPR Reader*, 50–56. Cambridge: Policy Press.

Graham, J., Nosek, B. A., Haidt, J., Iyer, R., Koleva, S. and Ditto, P. H. (2011). Mapping the moral domain. *Journal of personality and social psychology*, 101(2), 366.

Grant, R. W. (2002). The ethics of incentives: Historical origins and contemporary understandings. *Economics & Philosophy*, 18(1), 111–139.

Grant, R. W. (2006). Ethics and incentives: A political approach. *American Political Science Review*, 100(1), 29–39.

Grant, R. W. (2012). *Strings Attached: Untangling the Ethics of Incentives*. Princeton, NJ: Princeton University Press.

Gray, J. (2000). Inclusion: A radical critique, in Askonas, P. and Stewart, A. (eds) *Social Inclusion: Possibilities and Tensions*, 19–36. Basingstoke: Macmillan.

Greener, I. (2002). Agency, social theory and social policy. *Critical Social Policy*, 22(4), 688–705.

Greenhalgh, S. and Moss, J. (2009). *Principles for Social Housing Reform*. London: Localis.

Greer, P. and Horst, C. (2014). *Mission Drift: The Unspoken Crisis Facing Leaders, Charities, and Churches*. Bloomington, MA: Bethany House.

Gregg, P. and Tominey, E. (2005). The wage scar from male youth unemployment. *Labour Economics*, 12(4), 487–509.

Gregg, P., Harkness, S. and Macmillan, L. (2006). *Welfare to Work Policies and Child Poverty: A Review of Issues Relating to the Labour Market and Economy*. York: Joseph Rowntree Foundation.

Gregory, J. (2015). Engineering compassion: The institutional structure of virtue. *Journal of Social Policy*, 44(2), 339–356.

Griggs, J. and Evans, M. (2010). *Sanctions within Conditional Benefit Systems: A Review of Evidence*. York: Joseph Rowntree Foundation.

Grogger, J. and Karoly, L. (2005). *Welfare Reform: The Effects of a Decade of Change*. Cambridge, MA: Harvard University Press.

Grosh, M. E., del Ninno, C., Tesliuc, E. and Oeughi, A. (2008). *For Protection and Promotion: The Design and Implementation of Effective Safety Nets*. Washington, DC: World Bank.

Grover, C. (2010). Social security policy and vindictiveness. *Sociological Research Online*, 15(2), 8. www.socresonline.org.uk/15/2/8.html

Gugushvili, D. and Hirsch, D. (2014). *Means-testing or Universalism: What Strategies Best Address Poverty? A Review Contributing to Joseph Rowntree Foundation's Development of an Anti-poverty Strategy*. Loughborough: Centre for Research in Social Policy, Loughborough University.

Haidt, J. and Graham, J. (2007). When morality opposes justice: Conservatives have moral intuitions that liberals may not recognize. *Social Justice Research*, 20(1), 98–116.

Halpern, D., Bates, C., Mulgan, G., Aldridge, S., Beales, G. and Heathfield, A. (2004). *Personal Responsibility and Changing Behaviour: The State of Knowledge and its Implications for Public Policy*. London: Cabinet Office, Strategy Unit.

Handberg, R. (1980). Law, coercion, and incentives: Reconciling the irreconcilable, in Brigham, J. and Brown, D. (eds) *Policy Implementation: Penalties Or Incentives?* 103–112. Thousand Oaks, CA: Sage.

Hansen Lofstrand, C. (2010). Reforming the work to combat long-term homelessness in Sweden. *Acta Sociologica*, 53, 19–34.

Harford, T. (2008). *The Logic of Life: Uncovering the New Economics of Everything*. London: Little Brown.

Hastings, A., Bailey, N., Gannon, M., Besemer, K. and Bramley, G. (2015). Coping with the cuts? The management of the worst financial settlement in living memory. *Local Government Studies*, 41(4), 601–621.

Hausman, D. M. and Welch, B. (2010). Debate: To nudge or not to nudge. *Journal of Political Philosophy*, 18(1), 123–136.

Haux, T. (2013). Lone parents and activation – towards a typology of approaches. *Journal of International and Comparative Social Policy*, 29(2), 122–133.

Hay, C. (2004). Theory, stylized heuristic or Self-fulfilling prophecy? The status of rational choice theory in public administration. *Public Administration*, 82(1), 39–62.

Hayden, C. and Blaya, C. (2005). Children on the margins. *Policy Studies*, 26(1), 67–83.

Hern, A. (2013). Workfare ruled illegal, but only on narrow terms. *New Statesman*, 12th February. www.newstatesman.com/politics/2013/02/workfare-ruled-illegal-only-narrow-terms

Higgins, J. (1980). Social control theories of social policy. *Journal of Social Policy*, 9(1), 1–23.

Hill, M. (2014). Better to please the coroner than the auditor: Social policy delivery in challenging times, in Fransworth, L., Irving, Z. and Fenger, M. (eds) *Social Policy Review* 26, 103–118. Bristol: Policy Press.

Hills, J. (2013). *Labour's Record on Cash Transfers, Poverty, Inequality and the Lifecycle 1997 – 2010, Social Policy in a Cold Climate, Working Paper 5*. London: Centre for Analysis of Social Exclusion, London School of Economics.

Hills, J. (2014). *Good Times, Bad Times: The Welfare Myth of Them and Us*. Bristol: Policy Press.

Hirschi, T. and Gottfredson, M. R. (2005). Punishment of children from the perspective of control theory, in Donnelly, M. and Straus, M. (eds) *Corporal Punishment of Children in Theoretical Perspective*, 214–222. New Haven, CT: Yale University Press.

Hirschl, R. (2007). *Towards Juristocracy: The Origins and Consequences of the New Constitutionalism*. Cambridge, MA: Harvard University Press.

HM Treasury. (2015). Government announces Child Benefit deductions in tougher approach to truancy. *HM Treasury*, 6th October. www.gov.uk/government/news/government-announces-child-benefit-deductions-in-tougher-approach-to-truancy

Hofmann, B. (2008). *Work Incentives? Ex-post Effects of Unemployment Sanctions: Evidence from West Germany. IAB Discussion Paper 43/2008*. Nuremburg: IAB.

Hoggett, P. (2001). Agency, rationality and social policy. *Journal of Social Policy*, 30(1), 37–56.

Hoggett, P. (2006). Conflict, ambivalence, and the contested purpose of public organizations. *Human Relations*, 59(2), 175–194.

Hoggett, P., Wilkinson, H. and Beedell, P. (2013). Fairness and the politics of resentment. *Journal of Social Policy*, 42(3), 567–585.

Hood, A. and Waters, T. (2017a). *Living Standards, Poverty and Inequality in the UK: 2016–17 to 2021–22*. London: Institute for Fiscal Studies.

Hood, A. and Waters, T. (2017b). *The Impact of Tax and Benefit Reforms on Household Incomes. Briefing Note (BN196)*. London: IFS.

Horwitz, A. V. (1990). *The Logic of Social Control*. New York, NY: Plenum Press.

Hough, J., Jones, A. and Lewis, H. (2011). *No Second Night Out: An Evaluation of the First Six Months of the Project*. London: Broadway, University of York and Crunch Consulting.

House of Commons Work and Pensions Committee. (2017). Employment opportunities for young people. Ninth report of Session 2016–17. https://publications.parliament.uk/pa/cm201617/cmselect/cmworpen/586/586.pdf

Hudson, J. and Lowe, S. (2009). *Understanding the Policy Process: Analysing Welfare Policy and Practice*. Bristol: Policy Press.

Hudson, J., Lunt, N., Hamilton, C., Mackinder, S., Meers, J. and Swift, C. (2016). Exploring public attitudes to welfare over the Longue Durée: Re-examination of survey evidence from Beveridge, Beatlemania, Blair and Beyond. *Social Policy and Administration*, 50(6), 691–711.

Hultqvist, S. and Nørup, I. (2017). Consequences of activation policy targeting young adults with health-related problems in Sweden and Denmark. *Journal of Poverty and Social Justice*, 25(2), 147–161.

Humpage, L. (2016). Income management in New Zealand and Australia: Differently framed but similarly problematic for Indigenous peoples. *Critical Social Policy*, 36(4), 551–571.

Ignatieff, M. (2000). *I. Human Rights as Politics; II. Human Rights as Idolatry. Paper Presented at the Tanner Lectures on Human Values*. Princeton, NJ: Princeton University.

Jacobi, L. and Kluve, J. (2007). Before and after the Hartz reforms: The performance of active labour market policy in Germany. *Journal for Labour Market Research*, 40(1), 45–64.

Jacques, S. and Allen, A. (2013). Bentham's sanction typology and restrictive deterrence: A study of young, suburban, middle-class drug dealers. *Journal of Drug Issues*, 44(2), 212–230.

Jenks, C. (2003). *Transgression (Key Ideas)*. London: Routledge.

Jensen, P., Rosholm, M. and Svarer, M. (2003). The response of youth unemployment to benefits, incentives, and sanctions. *European Journal of Political Economy*, 19(2), 301–316.

Jewell, C. J. (2007). *Agents of the Welfare State. How Caseworkers Respond to Need in the United States, Germany, and Sweden*. New York, NY: Palgrave Macmillan.

Jochelson, K. (2007). *Paying the Patient: Improving Health Using Financial Incentives*. London: King's Fund.

John, P., Smith, G. and Stoker, G. (2009). Nudge nudge, think think: Two strategies for changing civic behaviour. *The Political Quarterly*, 80(3), 361–370.

Johnsen, S. (2014). Where's the 'faith' in 'faith-based' organisations? The evolution and practice of faith-based homelessness services in the UK. *Journal of Social Policy*, 43(2), 413–430.

Johnsen, S. (2016). *First Wave Findings: Lone Parents. Welfare Conditionality: Sanctions, Support and Behaviour Change*. York: University of York.

Johnsen, S. and Fitzpatrick, S. (2007). *The Impact of Enforcement on Street Users in England*. Bristol: Policy Press.

Johnsen, S. and Fitzpatrick, S. (2010). Revanchist sanitisation or coercive care? The use of enforcement to combat begging, street drinking and rough sleeping in England. *Urban Studies*, 47(8), 1703–1723.

Johnsen, S. and Jones, A. (2015). *The Reconnection of Rough Sleepers within the UK: An Evaluation.* London: Crisis.

Johnsen, S. and Teixeira, L. (2010). *Staircases, Elevators and Cycles of Change: 'Housing First' and Other Housing Models for Homeless People with Complex Support Needs.* London: Crisis.

Johnsen, S., Fitzpatrick, S. and Watts, B. (2018). Homelessness and social control: A typology. *Housing Studies*, DOI: 10.1080/02673037.2017.1421912.

Johnsen, S., Watts, B. and Fitzpatrick, S. (2016). *First Wave Findings: Homelessness. Welfare Conditionality: Sanctions, Support and Behaviour Change.* York: University of York.

Johnsen, S., Watts, B. and Fitzpatrick, S. (under review). Rebalancing the rhetoric? Normative stances regarding enforcement in street homelessness policy. Urban Studies.

Johnston, D. (2011). *A Brief History of Justice.* Chichester: Wiley-Blackwell.

Jones, A. and Pleace, N. (2010). *A Review of Single Homelessness in the UK 2000–2010.* London: Crisis.

Jones, K., Brown, J. and Bradshaw, J. (1978). *Issues in Social Policy.* London: Routledge and Kegan Paul.

Jones, R., Pykett, J. and Whitehead, M. (2013). *Changing Behaviours: On the Rise of the Psychological State.* Cheltenham: Edward Elgar Publishing.

Joseph Rowntree Foundation. (2016). *UK Poverty: Causes, Costs and Solutions.* York: Joseph Rowntree Foundation.

Joyce, L., Durham, J., Williams, M. and White, C. (2005). *Evaluation of Basic Skills Mandatory Training Pilot and National Enhancements: Interim Report. Department for Work and Pensions, Research Report No. 307.* Norwich: Her Majesty's Stationery Office.

Kabeer, N., Piza, C. and Taylor, L. (2012). *What are the Economic Impacts of Conditional Cash Transfer Programmes? A Systematic Review of the Evidence. Technical Report.* London: EPPI-Centre, Social Science Research Unit, Institute of Education, University of London.

Kahneman, D. and Tversky, A. (1979). Prospect theory: An analysis of decision under risk. *Econometrica: Journal of the Econometric Society*, 47(2), 263–291.

Keane, C., Callan, T., Savage, M., Walsh, J. R. and Colgan, B. (2014). Distributional impact of tax, welfare and public service pay policies: Budget 2015 and Budgets 2009–2015. *Quarterly Economic Commentary*, 43, 43–56.

Kenna, P. and M. Uhry. (2006). *How the Right to Housing Became Justiciable in France.* Brussels: FEANTSA.

Kenworthy, L. (2011). *Progress for the Poor.* Oxford: Oxford University Press.

Kersbergen, K., Vis, B. and Hemerijck, A. (2014). The great recession and welfare state reform: Is retrenchment really the only game left in town? *Social Policy and Administration*, 48(7), 883–904.

Keune, M. and Serrano, A. (2013). *Deconstructing Flexicurity: Alternative Perspectives*. London: Routledge.

Kidd, S. (2016). To condition or not to condition: What is the evidence? *Pathways' Perspectives on Social Policy in International Development*, 20. www.developmentpathways.co.uk/resources/to-condition-or-not-to-condition-what-is-the-evidence

King, D. (1999). *In the Name of Liberalism: Illiberal Social Policy in the USA and Britain*. Oxford: Oxford University Press.

King, J. (2012). *Judging Social Rights*. Cambridge: Cambridge University Press.

King, P. (2003). Housing as a freedom right. *Housing Studies*, 18(5), 661–672.

King, P. (2006). What do we mean by responsibility? The case of UK housing benefit reform. *Journal of Housing and the Built Environment*, 21 (2), 111–125.

King, P. (2011). Using big ideas: The application of political philosophy in housing research. *Housing, Theory and Society*, 28(2), 109–122.

Kintrea, K. (2006). *Having it All? Housing Reform Under Devolution, Housing Studies*. www.tandfonline.com/DOI/ref/10.1080/02673030500491732?scroll=top

Klein, C. and Hansen, L. A. (2016). *Balancing Inclusiveness, Work Incentives and Sustainability in Denmark. OECD Economic Department Working Papers No. 1338*. Paris: OECD Publishing.

Knotz, C. and Nelson, M. (2013). Quantifying 'conditionality': A new database on conditions and sanctions for unemployment benefit claimants. Paper prepared for the ESPANet conference, Poznan, September 5–7.

Korpi, W. and Palme, J. (1998). The paradox of redistribution and strategies of equality: Welfare state institutions, inequality, and poverty in the Western countries. *American Sociological Review*, 63(5), 661–687.

Kremer, M. (2016). Earned citizenship: Labour migrants' views on the welfare state. *Journal of Social Policy*, 45(3), 395–415.

Kristjánsson, K. (2002). *Justifying Emotions: Pride and Jealousy*. London: Routledge.

Kristjánsson, K. (2005). A utilitarian justification of desert in distributive justice. *Journal of Moral Philosophy*, 2(2), 147–170.

Kymlicka, W. (2002). *Contemporary Political Philosophy: An Introduction*. Oxford: Oxford University Press.

Lalive, R., van Ours, J. C. and Zweimuller, J. (2002). *The Effect of Benefit Sanctions on the Duration of Unemployment. IZA Discussion Paper No. 469*. Bonn: Institute for the Study of Labor (IZA).

Lambert, M. (2016). In pursuit of 'the welfare trait': Recycling deprivation and reproducing depravation in historical context. *People, Place and Policy*, 10(3), 225–238.

Lambie-Mumford, H. (2014). *Food Bank Provision and Welfare Reform in the UK*. Sheffield: Sheffield Political Economy Research Institute.

Lambie-Mumford, H. (2017). *Hungry Britain: The Rise of Food Charity*. Bristol: Policy Press.

Langenbucher, K. (2015). *How Demanding are Eligibility Criteria for Unemployment Benefits, Quantitative Indicators for OECD and EU Countries. OECD Social, Employment and Migration Working Papers, No. 166*. Paris: OECD Publishing.

Larsen, C. A. (2006). *The Institutional Logic of Welfare Attitudes: How Welfare Regimes Influence Public Support*. Aldershot: Ashgate Publishing Company.

Larsen, F. (2013). Active labor market reform in Denmark: The role of governance in policy change, in Brodkin, E. Z. and Marston, G. (eds) *Work and the Welfare State: Street-Level Organizations and Workfare Politics*, 103–123. Washington, DC: Georgetown University Press.

Le Grand, J. (1997). Knights, knaves or pawns? Human behaviour and social policy. *Journal of Social Policy*, 26(2), 149–169.

Lee, B. J., Slack, K. S. and Lewis, D. A. (2004). Are welfare sanctions working as intended? Welfare receipt, work activity and material hardship amongst TANF recipients. *Social Service Review*, 78(3), 370–403.

Lens, V. (2008). Welfare and work sanctions: Examining discretion on the front lines. *Social Service Review*, 82(2), 197–222.

Lévy Vroelant, C. and Reinprecht, C. (2014). Housing the poor in Paris and Vienna: The changing understanding of the 'social', in Scanlon, K., Whitehead, C. and Fernández Arrigoitia, M. (eds) *Social Housing in Europe*, 297–313. Chichester: John Wiley and Sons.

Lindhorst, T. and Mancoske, R. J. (2006). The social and economic impact of sanctions and time limits on recipients of temporary assistance to needy families. *Journal of Sociology and Social Welfare*, 33(1), 93–114.

Lindsay, C., Mcquaid, R. W. and Dutton, M. (2007). New approaches to employability in the UK: Combining 'Human Capital Development' and 'Work First' strategies? *Journal of Social Policy*, 36(4), 539–560.

Link, B. G. and Phelan, J. C. (2001). Conceptualizing stigma. *Annual Review of Sociology*, 27, 363–385.

Lipsky, M. (1980/2010). *Street-level Bureaucracy: Dilemmas of the Individual in Public Service*. New York, NY: Russell Sage Foundation.

Lister, R. (1996). Introduction: In search of the 'underclass', in Lister, R. (ed) *Charles Murray and the Underclass: The Developing Debate*, 1–16. London: IEA Health and Welfare Unit.

Lister, R. (2004). *Poverty*. Cambridge: Polity Press.

Loopstra, R., Reeves, A., McKee, M. and Stuckler, D. (2015a). *Do Punitive Approaches to Unemployment Benefit Recipients Increase Welfare*

*Exit and Employment? A Cross Area Analysis of UK Sanctioning Reforms. University of Oxford Sociology Working Papers, 2015-01.* Oxford: University of Oxford.

Loopstra, R., Reeves, A., Taylor-Robinson, D., Barr, B., McKee, M. and Stuckler, D. (2015b). Austerity, sanctions, and the rise of food banks in the UK. *BMJ (Clinical Research ed)*, 350, h1775.

Loveland, I. (1992). Square pegs, round holes: The 'right' to council housing in the post-war era. *Journal of Law and Society*, 19(3), 339–364.

Lukes, S. (2005). *Power: A Radical View*. Basingstoke: Palgrave Macmillan.

Lukes, S. (2008). *Moral Relativism*. London: Profile.

Lupton, R. with Burchardt, T., Fitzgerald, A., Hills, J., McKnight, A., Obolenskaya, P., Stewart, K., Thomson, S., Tunstall, R. and Vizard, P. (2015). *The Coalition's Social Policy Record: Policy, Spending and Outcomes 2010–2015*. London: London School of Economics.

Mabbett, D. (2005). The development of rights-based social policy in the European Union: The example of disability rights. *Journal of Common Market Studies*, 43(1), 97–120.

MacAskill, W. (2015). *Doing Good Better: Effective Altruism and a Radical Way to Make a Difference*. New Haven, CT: Yale University Press.

MacDonald, R. (ed) (1997). *Youth, the 'Underclass' and Social Exclusion*. London: Routledge.

Machin, S. and Marie, O. (2004). *Crime and Benefit Sanctions. CEP Discussion Paper No. 645*. London: Centre for Economic Performance, London School of Economics.

MacIntyre, A. (1981/2007). *After Virtue*. London: Duckworth and Co.

Mackie, P., Thomas, I. and Bibbings, J. (2017). Homelessness prevention: Reflecting on a year of pioneering Welsh legislation in practice. *European Journal of Homelessness*, 11(1), 81–107.

Marchal, S., Marx, I. and Van Mechelen, N. (2014). The great wake-up call? Social citizenship and minimum income provisions in Europe in times of crisis. *Journal of Social Policy*, 43(2), 247–267.

Marmot, M. (2005). Social determinants of health inequalities. *Lancet*, 365(9464), 1099–1104.

Marshall, T. H. (1950). *Citizenship and Social Class: And Other Essays*. Cambridge: Cambridge University Press.

Marteau, T. M., Ogilvie, D., Roland, M., Suhrcke, M. and Kelly, M. P. (2011). Judging nudging: Can nudging improve population health. *BMJ*, 342, d228.

McKnight, A. (2005). Employment: Tackling poverty through 'work for those who can', in Hills, J. and Stewart, K. (eds) *A More Equal Society? New Labour, Poverty, Inequality and Exclusion*, 23–46. Bristol: Policy Press.

McVicar, D. (2008). Job search monitoring intensity, unemployment exit and job entry: Quasiexperimental evidence from the UK. *Labour Economics*, 15(6), 1451–1468.

McVicar, D. (2010). Does job search monitoring intensity affect unemployment? Evidence from Northern Ireland. *Economica*, 77, 296–313.

McVicar, D. (2014). The impact of monitoring and sanctioning on unemployment exit and job-finding rates. *IZA World of Labor*, 49, 1–10. DOI: 10.15185/izawol.49

Mead, L. (1986). *Beyond Entitlement: The Social Obligations of Citizenship*. New York, NY: Free Press.

Mead, L. (1992). *The New Politics of Poverty*. New York, NY: Basic Books.

Mead, L. (1997). *The New Paternalism*. Washington, DC: Brookings Institution Press.

Mead, L. (2005). Welfare reform and citizenship, in Mead, L. M. and Beem, C. (eds) *Welfare Reform and Political Theory*, 172–199. New York, NY: Russell Sage Foundation.

Mead, L. (2011). *Expanding Work Programs for Poor Men*. Washington, DC: AEI Press.

Mead, L. (2014). Open letter in response to Policy Exchange report 'Smarter sanctions: Sorting out the system' by Guy Miscampbell, published 3 March 2014. Available at: www.welfareconditionality.ac.uk/share-your-views

Meers, J. (2014). 'Shifting the place of social security': The 'bedroom tax', discrimination and discretionary housing payments. *Journal of Social Welfare and Family Law*, 36(1), 85–87.

Meers, J. (2017). The bedroom tax in the Supreme Court: Implications of the judgment. *Journal of Poverty and Social Justice*, 25(2), 181–187.

Meyer, H. D. and Benavot, A. (eds) (2013). *PISA, Power, and Policy: The Emergence of Global Educational Governance*. Oxford: Symposium Books.

Midgley, J. (2016). Perspectives on responsibility in practice as revealed through food provisioning offers for rough sleepers. *Critical Social Policy*, 36(4), 610–629.

Milbourne, L. and Cushman, M. (2015). Complying, transforming or resisting in the new austerity? Realigning social welfare and independent action among English voluntary organisations. *Journal of Social Policy*, 44(3), 463–485.

Miller, D. (1992). Distributive justice: What the people think. *Ethics*, 102(3), 555–593.

Miller, D. (1999). *Principles of Social Justice*. Cambridge MA: Harvard University Press.

Mirrlees, J. A. (2010). *Dimensions of Tax Design: The Mirrlees Review*. Oxford: Oxford University Press.

Miscampbell, G. (2014). *Smarter Sanctions: Sorting out the System*. London: Policy Exchange.

Misetics, B. (2013). Criminalisation of homelessness in Hungary, in Fernandez Evangelista, G. and Jones, S. (eds) *Mean Streets: A Report on the Criminalisation of Homelessness in Europe*, 102–111. Brussels: L'Imprimerie Chauveheid.

Mitchell, D. (1997). The annihilation of space by law: The roots and implications of anti-homelessness laws in the United States. *Antipode*, 29, 303–336.

Moffitt, R. (2003). The role of non-financial factors in exit and entry in TANF. *Journal of Human Resources*, 38(supplement), 1221–1254.

Moffitt, R. (2008). *Welfare Reform: The US Experience Institute for Research on Poverty. Institute for Research on Poverty Discussion Paper No. 1334-08*. Madison, WI: Institute for Research on Poverty.

Morgan, J. (2010). Family intervention tenancies: The de (marginalisation). of social tenants? *Journal of Social Welfare and Family Law*, 32(1), 37–46.

Mulhall, S. and Swift, A. (1996). *Liberals and Communitarians*. Oxford: Blackwell.

Mullainathan, S. and Shafir, E. (2014). *Scarcity: The New Science of Having Less and How It Defines Our Lives*. New York, NY: Picador.

Müller, K.-U. and Steiner, V. (2008). *Imposed Benefit Sanctions and the Unemployment to Employment Transition: The German Experience. IZA Discussion Paper No. 3483*. Bonn: Institute for the Study of Labor (IZA).

Murray, C. (1984). *Losing Ground: American Social Policy, 1950–1980*. New York, NY: Basic Books.

Murray, C. (1990). *The Emerging British Underclass*. London: Institute of Economic Affairs.

Murray, C. (1994). *Underclass: The Crisis Deepens*. London: Institute of Economic Affairs.

Murray, C. (1996). The emerging British underclass, in Murray, C. A., Lister, R. and Buckingham, A. (eds) *Charles Murray and the Underclass: The Developing Debate*, 24–53. London: IEA Health and Welfare Unit.

Narain, K. and Ettner, S. (2017). The impact of exceeding TANF time limits on the access to healthcare of low-income mothers. *Social Work in Public Health*, 32(7), 452–460.

National Audit Office. (2016). *Benefit Sanctions: Report by the Comptroller and Auditor General*. London: National Audit Office.

National Audit Office. (2017). *Homelessness: Report by the Comptroller and Auditor General*. London: National Audit Office.

National Law Center on Homelessness and Poverty (NLCHP). (2014). *No Safe Place: The Criminalization of Homelessness in U.S. Cities*. Washington, DC: NLCHP.

NCSL. (2017). *Drug Testing for Welfare Recipients and Public Assistance*. National Conference of State Legislatures. www.ncsl.org/research/human-services/drug-testing-and-public-assistance.aspx

New, B. (1999). Paternalism and public policy. *Economics and Philosophy*, 15(1), 63–83.

Nicholls, C. M. (2009). Agency, transgression and the causation of homelessness: A contextualised rational action analysis. *International Journal of Housing Policy*, 9(1), 69–84.

Nicholls, C. M. (2010). Housing, homelessness and capabilities. *Housing, Theory and Society*, 27(1), 23–41.

Norman, R. (1998). *The Moral Philosophers: An Introduction to Ethics*. Oxford: Oxford University Press.

Nozick, R. (1974). *Anarchy, State, and Utopia*. New York, NY: Basic Books.

Nussbaum M. C. (2000). *Women and Human Development: The Capabilities Approach*. Cambridge: Cambridge University Press.

O'Grady, T. (2017). How politicians created, rather than reacted to, negative public opinion on benefits. LSE British Politics and Policy blog, 7th November. http://blogs.lse.ac.uk/politicsandpolicy/public-opinion-towards-welfare/?utm_content=buffer8e26d&utm_medium=social&utm_source=twitter.com&utm_campaign=buffer

O'Malley, P. (2009). Theorizing fines. *Punishment and Society*, 11(1), 67–83.

O'Sullivan, E. (2012). Varieties of punitiveness in Europe: Homelessness and urban marginality. *European Journal of Homelessness*, 6(2), 69–97.

Oakley, M. (2014). *Independent Review of the Operation of Jobseeker's Allowance Sanctions Validated by the Jobseekers Act 2013*. London: Her Majesty's Stationery Office.

OECD. (2015). Compare your country: Benefits, taxes and wages. www.oecd.org/els/benefits-and-wages.htm

Office of Family Assistance (OFA). (2017). OFA 'Dear colleague' letter on rescinding guidance concerning waiver and expenditure authority under section 1115 of the Social Security Act. 30th August. www.acf.hhs.gov/ofa/resource/ofa-dear-colleague-letter-on-rescinding-guidance-concerning-waiver-and-expenditure-authority-under-section-1115-of-the-social

Oliver, A. (2013). From nudging to budging: Using behavioural economics to inform public sector policy. *Journal of Social Policy*, 42(4), 685–700.

Olsson, L. E. and Nordfeldt, M. (2008). Homelessness and the tertiary welfare system in Sweden: The role of welfare state and non-profit sector. *European Journal of Homelessness*, 2, 157–174.

Padgett, D. K. and Priyam, P. (2017). Pavement dwelling in Delhi, India: An ethnographic account of survival on the margins. *Human Organization*, 76(1), 73–81.

Padgett, D. K., Henwood, B. F. and Tsemberis, S. (2016). *Housing First: Ending Homelessness, Transforming Systems and Changing Lives*. New York, NY: Oxford University Press.

Painter, A. and Thoung, C. (2015). *Creative Citizen, Creative State: The Principled and Pragmatic Case for a Universal Basic Income*. London: RSA.
Paris, C., Williams, P. and Stimson, B. (1985). From public housing to welfare housing, *Australian Journal of Social Issues*, 20(2), 105–117.
Parrott, S. and Sherman, A. (2007). TANF's results are more mixed than is often understood. *Journal of Policy Analysis and Management*, 26(2), 374–381.
Parsell, C. (2011). Responding to people sleeping rough: Dilemmas and opportunities for social work. *Australian Social Work*, 64(3), 330–345.
Parsell, C. (2016). Surveillance in supportive housing: Intrusion or autonomy? *Urban Studies*, 53(15), 3189–3205.
Parsell, C. and Marston, G. (2016). Supportive housing: Justifiable paternalism? *Housing, Theory and Society*, 33(2), 195–216.
Parsell, C. and Watts, B. (2017). Charity and justice: A reflection on new forms of homelessness provision in Australia. *European Journal of Homelessness*, 11(2), 1–12.
Patrick, R. (2011). Disabling or enabling: The extension of work-related conditionality to disabled people. *Social Policy and Society*, 10(3), 309–320.
Patrick, R. (2012). Work as the primary 'duty'of the responsible citizen: A critique of this work-centric approach. *People, Place & Policy Online*, 6(1), 5–15.
Paul-Ebhohimhen, V. and Avenell, A. (2008). Systematic review of the use of financial incentives in treatments for obesity and overweight. *Obesity Review*, 9, 355–367.
Pavetti, L., Derr, M. and Hesketh, H. (2003). *Review of Sanction Policies and Research Studies: Final Literature Review. Report to the Department of Health and Human Services, Office of the Assistant Secretary for Planning and Evaluation.* Washington, DC: Mathematica Policy Research.
Paz-Fuchs, A. (2008). *Welfare to Work: Conditional Rights in Social Policy*. Oxford: Oxford University Press.
Peck, L. R. (2007). What are the effects of welfare sanction policies? Or, using propensity scores as a subgroup indicator to learn more from social experiments. *American Journal of Evaluation*, 28, 256–274.
Pellerano, L. and Barca, V. (2014). *Does One Size Fit All? The Conditions for Conditionality in Cash Transfers. Oxford Policy Management Working Paper.* Oxford: OPM.
Pemberton, S., Pantazis, C. and Hillyard, P. (2018). Poverty and social harm: Challenging discourses of risk, resilience and choice, in Bramley, G. and Bailey, N. (eds) *Poverty and Social Exclusion in the UK. Volume 2 – The Dimensions of Disadvantage*, 245–266. Bristol: Policy Press.
Pérez-Muñoz, C. (2017). What is wrong with testing welfare recipients for drug use? *Political Studies*, DOI: 10.1177/0032321717692166.
Perkins, A. (2016). *The Welfare Trait: How State Benefits Affect Personality*. London: Palgrave Macmillan.

Peters, M. and Joyce, L. (2006). *A Review of the JSA Sanctions Regime: Summary Research Findings. DWP Research Report No. 313*. London: DWP.

Petty, J. (2016). The London spikes controversy: Homelessness, urban securitisation and the question of 'hostile architecture'. *International Journal for Crime, Justice and Social Democracy*, 5(1), 67–81.

Phelan, J., Link, B. G., Moore, R. E. and Stueve, A. (1997). The stigma of homelessness: The impact of the label 'Homeless' on attitudes toward poor persons. *Social Psychology Quarterly*, 60(4), 323–337.

Phillips, D. L. (1993). *Looking Backward: A Critical Appraisal of Communitarian Thought*. Princeton, NJ: Princeton University Press.

Phillips, M. (2000). Welfare and the state. *Royal Institute of Philosophy Supplements*, 45, 105–120.

Phillips, R., Parsell, C., Seage, N. and Memmott, P. (2011). *Assertive Outreach*. Melbourne: Australian Housing and Urban Research Institute.

Phoenix, J. (2008). ASBOs and working women: A new revolving door? in Squires, P. (ed) *ASBO Nation: The Criminalisation of Nuisance*, 289–303. Bristol: Policy Press.

Pierson, C. and Humpage, L. (2016). Coming together or drifting apart? Income maintenance in Australia, New Zealand, and the United Kingdom. *Politics and Policy*, 44(2), 261–293.

Pinker, S. (2011). *The Better Angels of our Nature*. New York, NY: Viking.

Plant, R. (1998). Citizenship, rights, welfare, in Franklin, J. (ed) *Social Policy and Social Work: The IPPR Reader*, 57–72. Cambridge: Policy Press.

Potts, C. and Martin, L. (2013). Penal visions of homelessness and responsibilization in Belgium, in Fernandez Evangelista, G. and Jones, S. (eds) *Mean Streets: A Report on the Criminalisation of Homelessness in Europe*, 75–89. Brussels: L'Imprimerie Chauveheid.

Priemus, H., Kemp, P. A. and Varady, D. P. (2005). Housing vouchers in the United States, Great Britain, and the Netherlands: Current issues and future perspectives. *Housing Policy Debate*, 16(3–4), 575–609.

Productivity Commission. (2017). *Introducing Competition and Informed User Choice into Human Services: Reforms to Human Services, Draft Report*. Canberra: Australian Government Productivity Commission.

Public Law Project. (undated). *An Introduction to Judicial Review*. London: Public Law Project.

Raja, C. (2014). Working on welfare-to-work: Analysing the role of commitment devices in the success of sanctions policies. *The Public Sphere 2014*. http://publicspherejournal.com/wp-content/uploads/2017/06/2-Raja-Welfare.pdf

Rawls, J. (1971/1999). *A Theory of Justice*. Cambridge, MA: Harvard University Press.

Ray, K., Sissons, P., Jones, K. and Vegeris, S. (2014). *Employment, Pay and Poverty: Evidence and Policy Review*. York: Joseph Rowntree Foundation.

Rector, R. (2012). Obama's end run on welfare reform, part two: Dismantling workfare. *The Backgrounder*, 2731. www.heritage.org/welfare/report/obamas-end-run-welfare-reform-part-two-dismantling-workfare

Reeve, K. (2017). Welfare conditionality, benefit sanctions and homelessness in the UK: Ending the 'something for nothing culture' or punishing the poor? *Journal of Poverty and Social Justice*, 25(1), 65–78.

Reeves, A. and Loopstra, R. (2017). 'Set up to fail'? How welfare conditionality undermines citizenship for vulnerable groups. *Social Policy and Society*, 16(2), 327–338.

Robson, P. and Poustie, M. (1996). *Homeless People and the Law*. London: Butterworths/Planning Exchange.

Rodger, J. J. (2008). *Criminalising Social Policy: Anti-social Behaviour and Welfare in a De-civilised Society*. Cullompton: Willan Publishing.

Rosenberg, L., Derr, M., Pavetti, L., Asheer, S., Angus, M. H., Sattar, S. and Max, J. (2008). *A Study of States' TANF Diversion Programs*. Princeton, NJ: Mathematica Policy Research.

Rossel, C., Courtoisie, D. and Marsiglia, M. (2017). How could CCTs' conditionalities reinforce vulnerability? Non-compliers and policy implementation gaps in Uruguay's Family Allowances. *Development Policy Review*. DOI: 10.1111/dpr.12327

Ryan, F. (2015). Death has become a part of Britain's benefits system. *The Guardian*, 27th August. www.theguardian.com/commentisfree/2015/aug/27/death-britains-benefits-system-fit-for-work-safety-net

Sage, D. (2012). Fair conditions and fair consequences? Exploring New Labour, welfare contractualism and social attitudes. *Social Policy and Society*, 11(3), 359–373.

Sahlin, I. (2005). The staircase of transition: Survival through failure. *Innovation*, 18(2), 115–136.

Saltkjel, T. and Malmberg-Heimonen, I. (2016). Welfare generosity in Europe: A multi-level study of material deprivation and income poverty among disadvantaged groups. *Social Policy and Administration*, 51(7), 1287–1310.

Sanders, B. and Albanese, F. (2017). *An Examination of the Scale and Impact of Enforcement Interventions on Street Homeless People in England and Wales*. London: Crisis.

Scanlon, K., Fernández Arrigoitia, M. and Whitehead, C. M. (2015). Social housing in Europe. *European Policy Analysis*, 17, 1–12.

Schneider, A. and Ingram, H. (1990). Behavioral assumptions of policy tools. *The Journal of Politics*, 52(2), 510–529.

Schott, L. (2012). *An Introduction to TANF*. Washington, DC: Center on Budget and Policy Priorities.

Schram, S., Soss, J., Fording, R. C. and Houser, L. (2009). Deciding to discipline: Race, choice, and punishment at the frontlines of welfare reform. *American Sociological Review*, 74(3), 398–422.

Scoccia, D. (2008). In defense of hard paternalism. *Law and Philosophy*, 27(4), 351–381.

Scottish Government. (2013). *The Potential Impacts of Benefit Sanctions on Individuals and Households*. Edinburgh: Scottish Government.

Scruggs, L. and Allan, J. P. (2006). The material consequences of welfare states: Benefit generosity and absolute poverty in 16 OECD countries. *Comparative Political Studies*, 39(7), 880–904.

Sefton, T. and Sutherland, H. (2005). Inequality and poverty under New Labour, in Hills, J. and Stewart, L. (eds) *A More Equal Society? New Labour, Poverty and Exclusion*, 231–250. Bristol: Policy Press.

Selbourne, D. (1994). *The Principle of Duty*. London: Sinclair Stevenson.

Selznick, P. (1998). Social justice: A communitarian perspective, in Etzioni, A. (ed) *The Essential Communitarian Reader*, 61–72. Oxford: Rowman and Littlefield.

Sen, A. (1992). *Inequality Reexamined*. Oxford: Oxford University Press.

Sheehy-Skeffington, J. and Rea, J. (2017). *How Poverty Affects People's Decision-making Processes*. York: Joseph Rowntree Foundation.

Simon, H. A. (1957). *Models of Man: Social and Rational*. London: John Wiley and Sons.

Singer, P. (2015). *The Most Good You Can Do: How Effective Altruism is Changing Ideas about Living Ethically*. New Haven, CT: Yale University Press.

Smart, J. J. C. and Williams, B. (1973). *Utilitarianism: For and Against*. Cambridge: Cambridge University Press.

Smith, J. (2016). An analysis of the effect of compulsory voting on youth political apathy. Wales Institute of Social and Economic Research Blog, 15th November. http://blogs.cardiff.ac.uk/wiserd/2016/11/15/an-analysis-of-the-effect-of-compulsory-voting-on-youth-political-apathy

Smith, N. (1996). *The New Urban Frontier: Gentrification and the Revanchist City*. New York, NY: Routledge.

Social Mobility Commission. (2016). *State of the Nation Report on Social Mobility in Great Britain*. London: Her Majesty's Stationery Office.

Somerville, P. and Bengtsson, B. (2002). Constructionism, realism and housing theory. *Housing, Theory and Society*, 19(3–4), 121–136.

Sosenko, F., Livingstone, N. and Fitzpatrick, S. (2013). *Overview of Food Aid Provision in Scotland*. Edinburgh: Heriot-Watt University/Scottish Government.

Spicker, P. (1984). *Stigma and Social Welfare*. Beckenham: Croom Helm.

Spicker, P. (2005). Targeting, residual welfare and related concepts: Modes of operation in public policy. *Public Administration*, 83(2), 345–365.

Spurr, H. (2014). Food for thought. *Inside Housing*, 7th February. www.insidehousing.co.uk/insight/insight/food-for-thought6-38718

Standing, G. (2011). Behavioural conditionality: Why the nudges must be stopped–an opinion piece. *Journal of Poverty and Social Justice*, 19(1), 27–38.

Standing, G. (2017). *Basic Income: And How We Can Make It Happen*. London: Penguin.

State Government of Victoria. (2012). *Pathways to a Fair and Sustainable Social Housing System*. Melbourne: State Government of Victoria.

Staufenberg, J. and Stone, J. (2016). Revealed: The high street firms that used benefits claimants for free labour. *The Independent*, 30th July. www.independent.co.uk/news/uk/politics/benefits-department-for-work-and-pensions-mandatory-work-activity-government-major-companies-free-a7163646.html

Steiner, H. (1975). Individual liberty. *Proceedings of the Aristotelian Society*, 75, 33–50.

Stephens, M. (2008). The role of the social rented sector, in Fitzpatrick, S. and Stephens, M. (eds) *The Future of Social Housing*, 27–38. London: Shelter.

Stephens, M. and Fitzpatrick, S. (2007). Welfare regimes, housing systems and homelessness: How are they linked. *European Journal of Homelessness*, 1(1), 201–211.

Stephens, M. and Stephenson, A. (2016). Housing policy in the austerity age and beyond, in Fenger, M., Hudson, J. and Needham, C. (eds) *Social Policy Review 28*, 63–85. Bristol: Policy Press.

Stephens, M., Fitzpatrick, S. and Wallace, A. (2010). *Study on Housing Exclusion: Welfare Policies, Housing Provision and Labour Markets*. Brussels: European Commission.

Stewart, S. and Wright, S. (2014). *Conditionality Briefing: Unemployed People. Welfare Conditionality: Sanctions, Support and Behaviour Change*. York: University of York.

Stuart, F. (2014). From 'rabble management' to 'recovery management': Policing homelessness in marginal urban space. *Urban Studies*, 51(9), 1909–1925.

Sullivan, E. V., Harris, R. A. and Pfefferbaum, A. (2010). Alcohol's effects on brain and behavior. *Alcohol Research and Health*, 33(1–2), 127–143.

Svarer, M. (2007). *The Effect of Sanctions on the Job Findings Rate: Evidence from Denmark. IZA Discussion Paper No. 3015*. Bonn: Institute for the Study of Labor (IZA).

Swain, J. (2003). Beg to differ. *The Guardian*, 3rd September. www.theguardian.com/society/2003/sep/03/comment

Swain, J. (2015). Passion and outrage are essential but not enough, in Social Life (ed) *Chris Holmes: In Memory of His Life and Work*, 18–23. www.social-life.co/news/post/chris_holmes/

Taylor, D. R., Gray, M. and Stanton, D. (2016). New conditionality in Australian social security policy. *Australian Journal of Social Issues*, 51(1), 3–26.

Taylor-Gooby, P. (2005). *Attitudes to Social Justice*. London: Institute for Public Policy Research.

Terum, L. I., Torsvik, G. and Øverbye, E. (2017). Discrimination against ethnic minorities in activation programme? Evidence from a vignette experiment. *Journal of Social Policy*, 1–18. DOI: 10.1017/S0047279417000113.

Thaler, R. and Sunstein, C. (2008). *Nudge: Improving Decisions About Health, Wealth and Happiness*. New Haven, CT: Yale University Press.

Theodorou, N. and Johnsen, S. (2017). Homelessness and adverse childhood experience. *Homeless in Europe*, Winter, 4–7.

Thomas, M. (2016). Waiting period for young people to access income support: Budget review 2015–16 index. Parliament of Australia. www.aph.gov.au/About_Parliament/Parliamentary_Departments/Parliamentary_Library/pubs/rp/BudgetReview201516/IncomeSup

Tinson, A., Ayrton, C., Barker, K., Born, T. B., Aldridge, H. and Kenway, P. (2016). *Monitoring Poverty and Social Exclusion 2016*. York: Joseph Rowntree Foundation.

Titmuss R. M. (1958). The social division of welfare: Some reflections on the search for equity, reprinted in Alcock, P., Glennerster, H., Oakley, A. and Sinfield, A. (eds) (2001) *Welfare and Wellbeing: Richard Titmuss's Contribution to Social Policy*, 59–70. Bristol: Policy Press.

Titmuss R. M. (1968). *Commitment to Welfare*. London: Allen and Unwin.

Titmuss, R. M. (1970/1997). The gift relationship: From human blood to social policy, in Oakley, A. and Ashton, J. (eds) *The Gift Relationship: Expanded and Updated Edition*. New York, NY: New Press.

Tonnies, F. (1887/1955). *Community and Association*. London: Routledge and Paul.

Torgersen, U. (1987). Housing: The wobbly pillar under the welfare state. *Scandinavian Housing and Planning Research*, 4(sup 1), 116–126.

Tosi, A. (2007). Homelessness and the control of public space – criminalising the poor? *European Journal of Homelessness*, 1, 225–236.

Townsend, P. (1979). *Poverty in the United Kingdom: A Survey of Household Resources and Standards of Living, 1967–1969*. Harmondsworth: Penguin Books.

Tsemberis, S. (2010). *Housing First: The Pathways Model to End Homelessness for People with Mental Illness and Addiction*. Center City, MN: Hazelden.

Turner, B. (1993). Outline of a theory of human rights. *Sociology*, 27(3), 489–512.

Tversky, A. and Kahneman, D. (1974). Judgment under uncertainty: Heuristics and biases. *Science*, 185(4157), 1124–1131.

United Nations Development Programme (UNDP). (2000). *Human Development Report 2000*. New York, NY: Oxford University Press.

United States Interagency Council on Homelessness (USICH). (2012). Searching out solutions: Constructive alternatives to the criminalization of homelessness. www.usich.gov/tools-for-action/searching-out-solutions

US Department of Housing and Urban Development. (2013). *Worst Case Housing Needs 2011: Report to Congress*. Washington, DC: US Department of Housing and Urban Development, Office of Policy Development and Research.

Van den Berg, G. J., Uhlendorff, A. and Wolff, J. (2015). *Under Heavy Pressure: Intense Monitoring and Accumulation of Sanctions for Young Welfare Recipients in Germany. IAB Discussion Paper 34/2015*. Nuremberg: Institute for Employment Research.

Vis, B., Van Kersbergen, K. and Hylands, T. (2011). To what extent did the financial crisis intensify the pressure to reform the welfare state? *Social Policy and Administration*, 45(4), 338–353.

Wacquant, L. (2009). *Punishing the Poor: The Neoliberal Government of Social Insecurity*. Durham, NC: Duke University Press.

Wacquant, L. J. (1997). Three pernicious premises in the study of the American ghetto. *International Journal of Urban and Regional Research*, 21(2), 341–353.

Waldfogel, J. (2010). *Britain's War on Poverty*. New York, NY: Russell Sage Foundation.

Waldron, J. (1993). *Liberal Rights: Collected Papers*. Cambridge: Cambridge University Press.

Walker, R. (2005). *Social Security and Welfare: Concepts and Comparisons*. Maidenhead: Open University Press.

Walter, R. J., Viglione, J. and Tillyer, M. S. (2017). One strike to second chances: Using criminal backgrounds in admission decisions for assisted housing. *Housing Policy Debate*, 27(5), 734–750.

Wang, J. and Van Vliet, O. (2016). Social assistance and minimum income benefits: Benefit levels, replacement rates and policies across 26 OECD countries, 1990–2009. *European Journal of Social Security*, 18(4), 333–355.

Watson, S. (2015). Does welfare conditionality reduce democratic participation? *Comparative Political Studies*, 48(5), 645–686.

Watts, B. (2014). Homelessness, empowerment and self-reliance in Scotland and Ireland: The impact of legal rights to housing for homeless people. *Journal of Social Policy*, 43(4), 793–810.

Watts, B., Fitzpatrick, S. and Johnsen, S. (2017). Controlling homeless people? Power, interventionism and legitimacy. *Journal of Social Policy*, 47(2), 235–252. DOI: 10.1017/S0047279417000289.

Watts, B., Fitzpatrick, S., Bramley, G. and Watkins, D. (2014). *Welfare Sanctions and Conditionality in the UK*. York: Joseph Rowntree Foundation.

Webb, P. (2014). *Homeless Lives in American Cities: Interrogating Myth and Locating Community*. New York, NY: Palgrave Macmillan.

Webster, D. (2015a). Benefit sanctions: Britain's secret penal system. *Centre for Crime and Justice Studies*, 26th January. www.crimeandjustice.org.uk/resources/benefit-sanctions-britains-secret-penal-system

Webster, D. (2015b). *Briefing: The DWP's JSA/ESA Sanctions Statistics Release and Hardship Payments Ad Hoc Statistical Release, November 2015*. Glasgow: University of Glasgow.

Webster, D. (2017). *Briefing: Benefit Sanctions Statistics: JSA, ESA, Universal Credit and Income Support for Lone Parents, August 2017*. Glasgow: University of Glasgow.

Welshman, J. (2013). *Underclass: A History of the Excluded Since 1880*. Second edition. London: Bloomsbury.

White, S. (2003). *The Civic Minimum: On the Rights and Obligations of Economic Citizenship*. Oxford: Oxford University Press.

White, S. (2017). Should a minimum income be unconditional? in Civitarese Matteucci, S. and Halliday, S. (eds) *Social Rights in Europe in An Age of Austerity*, 181–196. Abingdon: Routledge.

Whiteford, M. (2010). Hot tea, dry toast and the responsibilisation of homeless people. *Social Policy and Society*, 9(2), 193–205.

Whitworth, A. and Griggs, J. (2013). Lone parents and welfare-to-work conditionality: Necessary, just, effective? *Ethics and Social Welfare*, 7(2), 124–140.

Wilcox, S., Perry, J., Stephens, M. and Williams, P. (2017). *UK Housing Review: 25th Anniversary Edition*. Coventry: Chartered Institute of Housing.

Wilkinson, R. G. (2005). *The Impact of Inequality: How to Make Sick Societies Healthier*. Abingdon: Routledge.

Wilson, W. and Barton, C. (2017). Allocating social housing (England). House of Commons Library Briefing Paper, Number 06397, 9th June 2017. http://researchbriefings.parliament.uk/ResearchBriefing/Summary/SN06397

Wilson, W. J. (1987). *The Truly Disadvantaged: The Inner City, the Underclass, and Public Policy*. Chicago, IL: University of Chicago Press.

Wilson, W. J. (1997). *When Work Disappears: The World of the New Working Poor*. New York, NY: Vintage.

Wincup, E. (2014). Thoroughfares, crossroads and cul-de-sacs: Drug testing of welfare recipients. *International Journal of Drug Policy*, 25(5), 1031–1037.

Woodhall-Melnik, J. R. and Dunn, J. R. (2016). A systematic review of outcomes associated with participation in Housing First programs. *Housing Studies*, 31(3), 287–304.

Woodiwiss, A. (2005). *Human Rights (Key Ideas)*. London: Routledge.

Wright, S. (2012). Welfare-to-work, agency and personal responsibility. *Journal of Social Policy*, 41(2), 309–328.

Wright, S. and Stewart, A. (2016). *First Wave Findings: Jobseekers. Welfare Conditionality: Sanctions, Support and Behaviour Change*. York: University of York.

Wright, S., Dwyer, P., McNeill, J. and Stewart, A. (2016). *First Wave Findings: Universal Credit. Welfare Conditionality: Sanctions, Support and Behaviour Change*. York: University of York.

Wu, C.-F. (2008). Severity, timing, and duration of welfare sanctions and the economic well-being of TANF families with children. *Children and Youth Services Review*, 30, 26–44.

Wu, C.-F., Cancian, M., Meyer, D. R. and Wallace, G. L. (2006). How do welfare sanctions work? *Social Work Research*, 30(1), 33–50.

Young, I. M. (1990). *Justice and the Politics of Difference*. Princeton, NJ: Princeton University Press.

# INDEX